ARTHRITIS: TYPES, TREATMENT AND PREVENTION

IMMUNOLOGY AND IMMUNE SYSTEM DISORDERS

Additional books in this series can be found on Nova's website
under the Series tab.

Additional E-books in this series can be found on Nova's website
under the E-book tab.

ARTHRITIS: TYPES, TREATMENT AND PREVENTION

MARC N. PELT
EDITOR

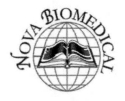

Nova Science Publishers, Inc.
New York

Arthritis : types, treatment, and prevention / editor, Marc N. Pelt.
    p. ; cm.
Includes bibliographical references and index.
ISBN 978-1-61470-719-6 (hardcover)
1. Arthritis--Chemotherapy. 2. Arthritis--Prevention. I. Pelt, Marc N.
[DNLM: 1. Arthritis--drug therapy. 2. Arthritis--prevention & control. WE 344]
RC933.A697 2011
616.7'2206--dc23
                        2011024681

Published by Nova Science Publishers, Inc. †*New York*

Contents

Preface

Osteoarthritis (OA) also known as degenerative arthritis or degenerative joint disease, is a group of mechanical abnormalities involving degradation of joints, including articular cartilage and subchondral bone. Symptoms may include joint pain, tenderness, stiffness, locking, and sometimes an effusion. Psoriatic arthritis is a type of inflammatory arthritis that will develop in up to 30 percent of people who have the chronic skin condition psoriasis. This book presents topical research on both these topics including the pharmacological treatment of osteoarthritis; the health effects and current treatment of psoriasis and psoriatic arthritis; the role of aquaporins in human synovitis and subclinical atherosclerosis in patients with psoriatic arthritis.

Chapter 1 - The pharmacological treatment of osteoarthritis (OA) has three goals: to relieve pain, to improve function and quality of life and to modify the course of the disease. Drugs targeting pain are analgesics, including opioid and non-opioid analgesics, oral or topical classical non-steroidal anti-inflammatory drugs, and selective cyclo-oxygenase-2 inhibitors (lumiracoxib, valdecoxib, etoricoxib, celecoxib). Chondroitin sulfate, glucosamine and diacerein showed efficacy in relieving pain and improving function in randomised trials, but meta-analyses showed conflicting results. Intra-articular corticosteroids and hyaluronans gave a variable relief from pain. The effect of medications on structural damage and course of the disease is questionable. Doxycycline, diacerein, chondroitin sulfate and glucozamine showed a beneficial effect on disease progression in randomised controlled trials (RCTs), but this effect is not invariably shown in meta-analyses. Cardiovascular safety concerns for NSAIDs have led to development of a cyclo-oxygenase-inhibiting, nitric oxide donor drugs (naproxcinod) that improved symptoms of OA, without adversely affecting blood pressure in

RCTs. A dual cyclo-oxygenase and 5-lipoxygenase inhibitor (licofelone), that decreases the production of pro-inflammatory prostaglandins and leukotrienes showed a symptomatic and chondroprotective effect, along with a favorable gastrointestinal safety profile. Disease-modifying antirheumatic drugs for rheumatoid arthritis are being studied in OA. These include methotrexate, hydroxychloroquine, and drugs targeting cytokines, such as interleukin-1 (anakinra, canakinumab) and tumor necrosis factor-α (infliximab, adalimumab). Biphosphonates, drugs that suppress osteoclasts and bone turnover, (risendronate and clodronate) showed contradictory effects on symptoms and radiographic progression in OA, while a bradykinin-receptor antagonist, icatibant, did not show any clear effect on pain. A novel, oral inhibitor of type-4 phosphodiesterase, apremilast, that has anti-inflammatory effects through downregulation of tumor necrosis factor-α, is being investigated in OA. Botulinum toxin type A is also under study as a pain relief medication for OA.

Chapter 2 - Psoriatic arthritis (PsA) types are described following the CLASsification of Psoriatic ARthritis (CASPAR) criteria, after the classic paper published by Moll and Wright in 1973. The PsA types can be summarized as: 1- Evidence of psoriasis (a) Current psoriatic skin or scalp disease (b) Personal history of psoriasis (c) Family history of psoriasis 2- Psoriatic nail dystrophy including onycholysis, pitting and hyperkeratosis 3 - A negative test for rheumatoid factor. 4 - Dactylitis 5 - Radiological evidence of juxta-articular new bone formation. A description of prevalence and incidence is presented, analyzing disease importance in the world. The relationship between psoriasis and PsA is analyzed from the genetic point of view. In psoriasis, the association is with class I antigens: HLAB13, HLA-B17, HLACw6, and HLA-Cw7. The allele HLA-Cw602 is associated with early onset of psoriasis, higher incidence of guttate or streptococcal induced disease flares, and more severe disease. The allele HLA-B27 is associated with greater spinal involvement, while B38 and B39 are associated with peripheral polyarthritis. In contrast to rheumatoid arthritis (RA), the joint distribution in PsA tends to be asymmetrical and oligoarticular (< five joints). Distal joints, particularly the distal interphalangeal (DIP) joints of the hands, are more frequently affected; joint tenderness tends to be less; and dactylitis, enthesitis and axial or spinal involvement are more frequent. PsA includes the absence of rheumatoid nodules, of rheumatoid factor in the blood and in some instances presence of iritis, mucous membrane lesions, urethritis, bowel inflammation and tendonitis. Patients with PsA have an increased incidence of cardiovascular disease (CVD) and cardiovascular risk factors such as smoking, hypertension, and metabolic syndrome compared to the normal population. In patients with PsA, carotid wave pulse velocity, a measure of arterial stiffness, is significantly higher as is subclinical atherosclerosis as measured by arterial intima-media wall thickness (IMT) and endothelial dysfunction. Therapies that target cells, such as activated T cells, and proinflammatory cytokines, such as tumor necrosis factor alpha (TNFα), are current treatments in use today. Traditional therapies for PsA like nonsteroidal anti-inflammatory drugs (NSAIDs), oral immunomodulatory drugs, topical creams, and light therapy have been helpful in controlling both musculoskeletal and dermatologic lesions of the disease, but may eventually show diminished benefit, and may produce severe toxicities as side effects. A first generation polyvalent vaccine, with leishmania amastigotes antigens, from 4 leishmania species has been found to decrease psoriasis and PsA, in several human clinical trials. Also mice collagen induced arthritis decreased markedly after treatment with purified leishmania antigens. Their antigenic effect has been explained by immunomodulation of T and B cells not by immunosuppression contrary to existing treatments on the market today.

Chapter 3 - Rheumatoid arthritis (RA) is an autoimmune disorder characterized by synovial proliferation (synovitis), articular cartilage and subchondral bone degradation and synovial inflammation. Joint swelling and oedema often accompany pannus formation and joint chronic inflammation in RA. Clinical evidence suggests that joint swelling and oedema frequently accompany the chronic inflammation observed in synovial joints of RA patients. Although joint swelling is understood to be a major problem in synovitis, very little is known about the molecular mechanisms responsible for the oedema fluid formation that is associated with joint inflammation. Recent studies from the authors' laboratory have shown that articular chondrocytes and synoviocytes express aquaporin 1 (AQP1) water channels. Aquaporins are a family of small integral membrane proteins related to the major intrinsic protein (MIP or AQP0). In recent studies the authors have used immunohistochemistry to investigate whether the expression of the AQP1 water channel is altered in synovitis. Their data suggests that this membrane protein is upregulated in the synovium derived from RA and psoriatic arthritis patients. In this chapter these observations are discussed in the context of RA and psoriatic arthritis. AQP1 and other aquaporins may play an important role in joint swelling and the vasogenic oedema fluid formation and hydrarthrosis associated with synovial inflammation.

Chapter 4 - Psoriasis is a multisystem disease with predominantly skin and joint manifestations, affecting 2% of the population. The proportion of patients with psoriasis who will develop psoriatic arthritis (PsA) ranges from 6% to 42% in different studies.

Not all therapies that target psoriasis however, can successfully treat PsA and vice versa.

The systemic agents – methotrexate, ciclosporin, leflunomide and numerous biologics can treat both skin and joint disease. Methotrexate decreases T and B cell function and suppresses cytokine secretion. Ciclosporin inhibits cytokine promoters with resultant decreased T-cell growth and migration. Leflunomide has both anti-proliferative and anti-inflammatory effects.

Biologics have now been increasingly used for patients with both psoriasis and PsA where first-line therapy has failed. A detailed work-up is necessary prior to initiation.

The first biological agents widely used for psoriasis and PsA are the TNF inhibitors comprising adalimumab, etanercept and infliximab. Adalimumab is the first fully human anti-TNF-α-monoclonal antibody. Etanercept is a recombinant human TNF-α receptor (p75) protein fused with the Fc portion of IgG1. Infliximab is a chimeric antibody comprising a mouse variable region and human IgG1-α constant region.

Golimumab is a newer monoclonal antibody, which binds to soluble and transmembrane forms of TNF-α. Improvements in PsA and skin disease have been reported in the large phase III multicenter, randomized, placebo-controlled study (Go-REVEAL). Certolizumab pegol (CDP 870) is a pegylated Fab fragment of a humanized anti-TNF-α antibody and in patients with moderate to severe plaque psoriasis, has shown results comparable with adalimumab and infliximab. So far, no phase III studies have been conducted for PsA patients.

Alefacept and efalizumab are T-cell modulators. Alefacept blocks the activation and proliferation of the key T-cells in psoriasis and aids granzyme-mediated apoptosis of T cells. Efalizumab has unfortunately been withdrawn from the market.

Newer agents in the therapeutic armamentarium are the anti-IL-12p40 antibodies: ustekinumab and briakinumab. Ustekinumab is a human immunoglobulin monoclonal antibody to the shared p40 subunit of IL-12 and IL-23. The effect of ustekinumab on cutaneous psoriasis appears to be at least comparable to or better than that of TNF inhibitors and is also promising for PsA. Briakinumab (ABT-874) is a recombinant, fully human IgG1 monoclonal antibody that binds to the same p40 subunit. Early studies have shown high efficacy in the treatment of psoriasis.

This chapter provides an overview of the concurrent treatment strategies for both the skin and joint manifestations of psoriasis

Chapter 5 - Osteoarthritis (OA), one of the most common joint diseases, is characterized by a slow degradation of cartilage over a long period. OA of the hip and knee causes chronic disability because of the related pain and functional impairment. Currently the most widely used treatment in OA is administration of nonsteroidal anti-inflammatory drugs (NSAIDs) from the early stages of the disease to relieve pain. However, although NSAIDs are useful for pain management, there are reports that they might accelerate progression of the disease. Intra-articular injections of high molecular weight hyaluronic acid (HA) are also used in the treatment of moderate-to-severe OA for pain relief and cartilage protection. HA is a major component of synovial fluid and plays a central role in joint lubrication; in OA, however, HA levels in the synovial fluid decrease. Several clinical trials have shown that intra-articular HA injections are effective and safe for OA patients who have ongoing pain and who are unable to tolerate other conservative treatments or joint replacement.

We examined the combination effects of intra-articular HA and oral NSAIDs on cartilage degeneration and onset of pain in a rabbit knee OA model. The rabbit OA model was made by partial meniscectomy. A NSAID was administered orally daily for 14 days, starting from the day of meniscectomy. HA was injected intra-articularly into the injured knee every 3 days from the day of surgery. The effect on pain was assessed by an incapacitance tester, and cartilage damage was evaluated by visual assessment and histopathology at 14 days after the surgery. Weight bearing on the injured hind paw decreased time-dependently in the control group. In the HA, NSAID, and HA+NSAID groups, this decrease in hind paw weight bearing was suppressed, demonstrating an analgesic effect. Visible damage and histopathological findings of cartilage degeneration were evident in the cartilages of the control group at day 14. In the HA group, the area of damaged cartilage decreased and cartilage degeneration was ameliorated. In contrast, in the NSAID group, surprisingly, the cartilage degeneration was exacerbated compared with the control group. The exacerbated cartilage degeneration induced by the NSAID was reversed by the concomitant use of HA. The levels of matrix metalloproteinases (MMP) -1, MMP-3, and MMP-13 in synovial fluid from the NSAID group were significantly higher than in controls. The increased production of MMPs induced by NSAIDs was counteracted by the concomitant administration of HA.

To analyze the phenomenon of MMP production in the rabbit OA model, the authors further studied the effects of HA and NSAIDs on the production of matrix metalloproteinases (MMPs) MMPs from human chondrocytes in vitro. Chondrocytes were cultured with an NSAID and HA in the presence of interleukin (IL)-1☐ or IL-6+sIL-6R for 24 h. After culture, the production of MMPs, IL-1☐, and IL-6 were measured. Their results clearly showed that HA inhibited NSAID-accelerated MMP production, which was followed by production of inflammatory cytokines from cytokine-activated chondrocytes. These results warrant further evaluation of the potential chondroprotective effects of co-administration of HA with NSAIDs.

There are many reports describing the biological activities of HA other than those deriving from its viscoelastic properties. HA has an inhibitory effect on IL-1- or lipopolysaccharide-induced production of inflammatory mediators. Overproduction of IL-6 was observed in OA synovial fluids; therefore, the authors investigated whether IL-6 induced MMP production. Moreover, they examined whether HA inhibits IL-6-induced MMP production and, if so how HA inhibits IL-6 signaling. Pre-treatment of cells with HA reduced IL-6-induced MMP production and the phosphorylation of extracellular-signal-regulated kinase (ERK). Expression levels of mitogen-activated protein kinase phosphatase (MKP-1), a negative regulator of ERK1/2, was increased in IL-6-treated chondrocytes. The authors' study was the first to demonstrate that HA suppressed induction of MMPs by IL-6 in human chondrocytes via induction of MKP-1.

The authors' study and other studies showed that the viscosupplementation and anti-inflammatory effects of HA are clearly involved in improving the symptoms of OA with a very favorable safety profile. Although current guidelines recommend the use of HA only after the unsuccessful use of NSAIDs, the authors demonstrated that concomitant use of HA is beneficial for reducing the adverse effects of NSAIDs. It is suggested that HA-based therapy from an earlier stage be recommended due to its role in preserving joint functions and maintaining the quality of life of OA patients

Chapter 6 - Accelerated development of atherosclerosis has been observed in patients with rheumatic diseases such as rheumatoid arthritis (RA) and psoriatic arthritis (PsA). It may be related to the inflammatory overload accompanied to the combination of an excessive production of reactive oxygen species with an impaired antioxidant defence capacity, leading to oxidative stress that may facilitate the development and progression of atherosclerosis.

Compared with the general population, patients with RA die prematurely, mainly because of cardiovascular diseases but the mechanism by which premature atherosclerosis develops in RA is unknown. Recent data have demonstrated the prevalence of atherosclerosis also in patients with PsA, a chronic inflammatory autoimmune disease characterized by inflammatory arthritis and skin psoriasis. PsA shares some phenotypic characteristics with RA, even though the synovial inflammation of PsA is characterized by less macrophage infiltration and increased vascularity in comparison to RA inflammation. The increased cardiovascular risk in PsA and RA suggests the need to treat the inflammatory process and to monitor traditional atherosclerotic risk factors in these pathologies.

The aim of the athors' study was to evaluate whether increased oxidative stress may be associated to the presence of subclinical atherosclerosis in patients with RA and in patients with PsA. For this purpose the authors determined the levels of oxidized low density lipoproteins (ox-LDL) and of nitric oxide (NO) in the sera obtained from 19 patients with RA, 20 with PsA and 20 sex- and age-matched healthy controls. Patients with RA fulfilled the American College of Rheumatology criteria, and patients with PsA fulfilled the CASPAR criteria. In all patients the authors evaluated the activity and duration of the disease and classical risk factors for atherosclerosis. Their results showed higher levels of ox-LDL and lower levels of NO in sera from patients with RA and PsA than in sera from healthy controls. Notably, higher serum levels of ox-LDL were observed in patients with an intima-media thickness (IMT) >1 than in those with an IMT ≤1, and higher serum levels of NO in patients with an IMT ≤1 than in those with an IMT >1, in patients with RA and PsA. The authors' data suggest that monitoring circulating levels of ox-LDL and NO in patients with RA and PsA could give information on the development of atherosclerotic disease and therefore could be useful to the clinical management of patients.

Chapter 7 - Arthrodesis of the wrist has been considered as the gold standard for osteoarthritis of the wrist. In 1984 Watson and Ballet [1] recognized a specific pattern of carpal collaps (SNAC), other alternatives have been proposed: the proximal row carpectomy (PRC) and the scaphoidectomy combined with a four corner arthrodesis. In this cohort of 54 patients, two motion preserving procedures were compared (26 PRC's and 28 four corner fusions). The PRC had significantly better outcome for range of motion and DASH. Grippping force was not significantly different between both procedures.

In: Arthritis: Types, Treatment and Prevention   ISBN 978-1-61470-719-6
Editor: Marc N. Pelt   © 2012 Nova Science Publishers, Inc.

Chapter I

The Pharmacological Treatment of Osteoarthritis

Athanasios Koutroumpas, Theodora Simopoulou and Lazaros I. Sakkas

Rheumatology Clinic
Medical School, Faculty of Health Sciences,
University of Thessalia, Greece

ABSTRACT

The pharmacological treatment of osteoarthritis (OA) has three goals: to relieve pain, to improve function and quality of life and to modify the course of the disease. Drugs targeting pain are analgesics, including opioid and non-opioid analgesics, oral or topical classical non-steroidal anti-inflammatory drugs, and selective cyclo-oxygenase-2 inhibitors (lumiracoxib, valdecoxib, etoricoxib, celecoxib). Chondroitin sulfate, glucosamine and diacerein showed efficacy in relieving pain and improving function in randomised trials, but meta-analyses showed conflicting results. Intra-articular corticosteroids and hyaluronans gave a variable relief from pain. The effect of medications on structural damage and course of the disease is questionable. Doxycycline, diacerein, chondroitin sulfate and glucozamine showed a beneficial effect on disease progression in randomised controlled trials (RCTs), but this effect is not invariably shown in meta-analyses. Cardiovascular safety concerns for NSAIDs have led to development of a cyclo-oxygenase-inhibiting, nitric oxide donor drugs (naproxcinod) that improved symptoms of OA, without adversely affecting blood pressure in RCTs. A dual cyclo-oxygenase and 5-lipoxygenase inhibitor (licofelone), that decreases the production of pro-inflammatory prostaglandins and leukotrienes showed a symptomatic and chondroprotective effect, along with a favorable gastrointestinal safety profile. Disease-modifying antirheumatic drugs for rheumatoid arthritis are being studied in OA. These include methotrexate, hydroxychloroquine, and drugs targeting cytokines, such as interleukin-1 (anakinra, canakinumab) and tumor necrosis factor-α (infliximab, adalimumab). Biphosphonates, drugs that suppress osteoclasts and bone turnover, (risendronate and clodronate) showed contradictory effects on symptoms and radiographic progression in OA, while a bradykinin-receptor antagonist, icatibant, did not show any clear effect on pain. A novel, oral inhibitor of type-4 phosphodiesterase, apremilast, that has anti-inflammatory effects through downregulation of tumor necrosis factor-α, is being investigated in OA. Botulinum toxin type A is also under study as a pain relief medication for OA.

INTRODUCTION

Osteoarthritis (OA) is the most common arthritis, affecting 13.9% of adult United States (US) population over age 25, and 33.6% of those over age 65 [Lawrence et al, 2008]. OA results in pain, loss of function, disability and a decline in quality of life [Guccione et al, 1994]. In younger individuals, OA has an impact on productivity and loss of hours from work [Buckwalter et al, 2004]. OA accounts for over half of arthritis-related hospitalizations [Lethbridge-Cejku et al, 2003] and 6% of all arthritis-related deaths in the USA [Sacks et al, 2004]. Taking into account the aging of the USA and Europe population, the economic and social impact of OA is expected to increase.

The treatment of OA is far from satisfactory. The discovery of new drugs for OA has been impeded for several reasons. OA is a condition of unknown etiology, and has a considerable heterogeneity. It has many pathological facets, such as cartilage degradation, subchondral sclerosis and cysts, new bone formation, erosive changes, synovitis, tenosynovitis, and ligament degeneration, and the contribution of each one to OA symptoms, function and progression is not fully understood. The lack of association between radiological, clinical and objective signs is another concern for study design and interpretation of results. OA is a very slowly progressing disease and requires long-term trials to reveal any disease-modifying properties of drugs under study. OA trials use more often various subjective, patient-oriented end points, and less often objective end-points, making comparison of results difficult. As a chronic, painful condition, overall patient-reported responses in OA may be influenced by unknown factors, as illustrated by the unusually high response rates seen in placebo groups [Zwang et al., 2008a]. Finally, methodological issues in OA trials and meta-analyses add further concerns [Nüesch et al., 2010; Nüesch et al., 2009a].

Treatment Goals

Ideally, an efficacious medication should alleviate symptoms, improve function, retard disease progression, or even promote healing of existing damage, with a reasonable safety. Thus, a drug for OA should show improvement of subjective, patient-reported outcomes for pain and function and show evidence of slowing radiographic damage [Hunter DJ, 2011; Abadie et al, 2004]. Radiographic progression is mainly expressed as change in joint space width in plain radiographs, which is used as a surrogate marker for cartilage thickness, and to a lesser degree as change in the number and size of osteophytes and subchondral bone sclerosis [Hunter et al, 2009]. More recent research uses magnetic resonance imaging (MRI) of the joint for a more accurate assessment of articular cartilage, synovium, ligaments, menisci, and subchondral bone. However, further validation is needed before MRI is used as an end-point for structure modifying drugs in OA [Hunter et al, 2009; Amin et al, 2005].

PHARMACOLOGICAL AGENTS IN OA

1. Analgesics

Simple analgesics are the first line of treatment for any symptomatic OA patient. Non-opioid analgesics, such as acetaminophen, can be used in doses up to 4 g per day, and is commonly used as the comparator drug in randomised controlled trials (RCTs) [Pincus et al, 2001; Batlle-Gualda et al, 2007; Temple et al, 2006]. A recent review assessed the efficacy of acetaminophen compared to placebo or non-steroidal anti-inflammatory drugs (NSAIDs) in RCTs. Acetaminophen was found to be slightly superior to placebo for pain. Short-term trials (for 6 weeks) found acetaminophen to be inferior to NSAIDs [Towheed et al, 2009]. The major advantage of acetaminophen is a favourable safety profile in doses up to 4 g per day [Zhang et al, 2004]. However, there may be an increased risk of gastrointestinal (GI) complaints in doses >2 g/day [Garcia Rodriguez et al, 2001]. These GI complaints are usually heartburn, abdominal discomfort and nausea, and rarely ulcers [Bannwarth B, 2004]. A bias is possible, since patients at increased risk for GI complications would be preferentially given acetaminophen over NSAIDs [Nickles et al, 2005]. Therefore, acetaminophen is considered a safe alternative for patients with contraindications or intolerant to NSAIDs and can also be used as an "NSAID sparing agent" for long-term use [Nickles et al, 2005].

Opioid preparations, such as oral codeine, morphine, oxycodone and oxymorphone and transdermal fentanyl and buprenorphine have shown effectiveness in relieving pain and improving function, irrespective of opioid type [Nüesch et al, 2009b].

The use of opioids in OA is limited by their frequent side effects. Common adverse events include nausea, somnolence, dizziness, vomiting and constipation. Serious events, such as respiratory depression, sedation and confusion are less frequent and can be limited with a slow dose titration [Pergolizzi et al, 2008]. A negative effect on balance that predispose to falls is of concern, especially in the elderly [Vestergaard et al, 2006]. Opioids may cause addiction in OA patients; a withdrawal syndrome has been described for transdermal fentanyl [Langford et al, 2006], and a review of 24 studies with 2,507 OA patients on opioids showed that addiction/abuse was seen in 3.3% of patients [Fishbain et al, 2008].

Tramadol, a weak μ-opioid agonist and serotonin-norepinephrine reuptake inhibitor has shown efficacy in reducing pain and improving function in OA in RCTs, but the size effect is small [Cepeda et al, 2006; Cepeda et al, 2007]. Tramadol can be used to reduce the dose of NSAIDs [Schnitzler et al, 1999]. Tramadol is also available in slow-release form and in a combination with acetaminophen.

Common adverse effects of tramadol, occurring in 25% of patients, are opioid-related and include nausea, constipation, sweating, dizziness and headache. A potential side effect, associated with its serotoninergic action, namely seizures, occurs in less than 1% [Gardner et al, 2000; Gasse et al, 2000]. Addiction/drug abuse is rare [WHO Expert Commitee on Drug Dependence, 2008]. Tramadol should be used cautiously with selective serotonin reuptake inhibitors, whereas co-administration of tramadol with monoamine oxidase inhibitors is contraindicated [Beaulieu et al, 2008].

2. Non-Steroidal Anti-Inflammatory Drugs

Non-steroidal anti-inflammatory drugs (NSAIDs) inhibit the cyclo-oxygenase (COX), thus inhibiting the production of prostaglandins (PGs), including PGE2, an important mediator of inflammation. There are two isoenzymes of COX, COX-1 and COX-2. COX-1 is constitutively expressed in most tissues, and its expression does not vary greatly, whereas COX-2 is over-expressed locally at the inflammation sites. NSAIDs inhibit COX-1 and – 2 to varying degrees. Thus, NSAIDs are divided into those that preferentially inhibit COX-2 ("selective COX-2 inhibitors"), and those that inhibit both COX-1 and COX-2 ("non-selective" COX inhibitors). This degree of inhibition is dependent on the concentration of the drug [FitzGerald and Patrono, 2001], which may show considerable variability after oral administration of the drug. Therefore, NSAIDs can be classified into those with high likelihood to spare COX-1 (lumiracoxib, etoricoxib and valdecoxib), intermediate (celecoxib, nimesulide, diclofenac and meloxicam) and low likelihood to spare COX-1 (naproxen, indomethacin and ibuprofen) [Patrono, 2007].

Table 1. Dosage of some commonly prescribed NSAIDs

Drug	Dosage
Aspirin	3 g/day, divided into 4-6 doses
Celecoxib	200 mg/day
Diclofenac	Delayed release: 100-150 mg/day in 2-3 doses Extended release: 100-200 mg/day
Etoricoxib	60 mg/day
Fenoprofen	300-600 mg, 3-4 times a day, max dose 3200 mg/day
Ibuprofen	1200-3200 mg/day, divided into 3-4 doses
Indomethacin	25-50 mg 2-3 times a day, max dose 200mg/day Extended release: 75 mg, 1-2 times a day
Ketoprofen	150-300 mg/day divided into 3-4 doses Extended release: 100-200 mg/day in a single dose
Meloxicam	7.5-15 mg/day, in a single dose
Naproxen	250-500 mg twice daily
Nimesulide	100 mg twice daily
Piroxicam	20 mg/day, in a single dose
Valdecoxib	10 mg/day, in a single dose

Growing evidence shows that NSAIDs improve pain and function in OA. Dosing of the most commonly used NSAIDs in OA is shown in Table 1. Efficacy has been shown for oral and topical preparations [Chou et al, 2006]. NSAIDs are modestly superior to acetaminophen, but due to safety considerations both the European League Against Rheumatism (EULAR) and Osteoarthritis Research Society International (OARSI) recommend the use of NSAIDs after a course of acetaminophen has failed to control symptoms [Zhang et al, 2005; Zhang et al, 2007; Jordan et al, 2003; Zhang et al, 2008a]. No clear superiority in efficacy has been shown for any NSAID [Chou et al, 2006], although an individual, non-predicted response can be seen, i.e., one NSAID efficacious for one patient may not be efficacious for another patient [Brooks and Day, 1991]. A course of 10 days is usually enough to assess the efficacy of a single NSAID in a particular patient [Brooks P, 1998].

Table 2. Adverse effects of NSAIDs

ADVERSE REACTIONS OF NSAIDs	
Gastrointestinal	Gastric mucosal irritation, erosions, ulcers Hemorrhage Nausea, vomiting, diarrhea, constipation Small bowel erosions Elevation of liver enzymes, hepatotoxicity
Renal	Acute renal failure, Decrease in glomerular filtration rate Interstitial nephritis Fluid retention
Cardiovascular	Hypertension Myocardial infarction
Central Nervous System	Headaches, strokes, tremor, depersonalization reactions, depression, hallucinations Aseptic meningitis, vertigo
Hematologic	Bone marrow suppression Decreased platelet aggregation
Hypersensitivity	Asthma, urticaria, angioedema, generalized pruritus, photosensitivity, Stevens-Jonson syndrome, toxic epidermal necrolysis

Other	pulmonary infiltrates with eosinophilia,
	Drug interactions
	   – warfarin, antiepileptics, lithium,
	   – diuretics, aminoglycosides, cyclosporine-A

A disease modifying effect has not been demonstrated for NSAIDs in OA. However, in ankylosing spondylitis (AS), long-term, continuous NSAID use has been associated with retardation of radiographic progression compared to on-demand use [Wanders et al, 2005]. Inhibition of COX-2 reduces callus formation after fracture in mice [Zhang et al, 2002] and NSAIDs are used for prevention of heterotopic ossification after hip replacement [Fransen and Neal, 2000].

From these results, the effect of long-term NSAID use on osteophyte formation might be expected to be favourable, but chondroprotective properties of NSAIDs in OA remain to be proved.

2.1. Adverse Effects

While the inhibition of PGE2 is crucial for the anti-inflammatory effects of NSAIDs, inhibition of prostacyclin (PGI2) in vascular endothelial cells and thromboxane (TXA2) (thromboxane) in platelets is responsible for adverse events. Adverse events of NSAIDs are listed in Table 2.

2.1.1. Gastrointestinal Adverse Effects

Gastrointestinal (GI) side effects are a major concern, and have led to the development of COX-2 selective inhibitors. Serious GI side effects are gastroduodenal ulcers and their complications, hemorrhage, perforation, and obstruction. GI adverse events are common; endoscopy-detected ulcers occur in up to 50% of NSAID-treated patients at 24 weeks [Patrono, 1998]. Risk factors for GI adverse effects are [Hernandez-Diaz and Garcia Rodriguez, 2001]:

- age > 65 years,
- history of peptic ulcer
- history of peptic hemorrhage,
- concomitant use of anticoagulants,
- concomitant use of cardioprotective aspirin,
- concomitant use of glucocorticosteroids,
- high dose of NSAID,
- use of different NSAIDs

Some 85% of patients with OA are considered to be high or moderate risk patients for GI complications [Lanas et al, 2010]. Selective COX-2 inhibitors reduce the risk for serious GI adverse effects by half [Schnitzer et al, 2004]. The use of a proton pump inhibitor (PPI) or misoprostol with an NSAID reduces the risk of symptomatic ulcer [Brown et al, 2006]. There is no evidence that H2-blockers or antacids prevent GI adverse effects [Hooper et al, 2004; Brown et al, 2006].

Although direct comparisons on the relative effectiveness of different gastroprotective strategies (COX-2 vs COX-1 plus PPI, COX-2 plus PPI vs COX-1 plus PPI) are lacking [Brown et al, 2006], addition of a PPI to either COX-2 selective inhibitor or non-selective NSAID is a cost-effective approach, even in patients with low risk for GI complications [Latimer et al, 2009]. For patients without any GI risk, all NSAIDs are appropriate. For patients with elevated GI risk, COX-2 selective inhibitors plus PPI or non selective NSAIDs plus PPI is recommended [Burmester et al, 2011].

2.1.2. Renal Adverse Effects

Renal adverse effects of NSAIDs, both non-selective and selective COX-2 inhibitors, include acute renal failure, interstitial nephritis, fluid retention and hypertension [Swan et al, 2000, Brater et al, 2001]. NSAID users have a 3-fold increased risk for acute renal failure [Huerta et al, 2005]. This risk is dose-dependent and is associated with both short- and long-term treatment. Risk factors for renal complications are [Huerta et al, 2005; Hernandez-Diaz and Garcia Rodriguez, 2001]:

- age >65 years,
- male gender,
- congestive heart failure
- concomitant use of diuretics,
- preexisting renal disease,
- hypo-albuninaemia,
- hypertension,
- diabetes mellitus

2.1.3. Cardiovascular Adverse Effects

Cardiovascular (CV) events associated with NSAIDs are a major concern. Since the original description of increased frequency of myocardial infarction in patients treated with the COX-2 inhibitor rofecoxib [Juni et al, 2004], many studies looked at the CV risk of non selective and selective COX-2 inhibitors. Selective COX-2 inhibitors are associated with a 40% increase in the frequency of serious vascular events, mainly myocardial infarction, whether on concomitant low-dose aspirin or not [Kearney et al, 2006]. A recent meta-analysis of 31 trials with more than 116.000 participants, assessing the CV risk of seven non-selective and selective COX-2 inhibitors concluded that all NSAIDs are associated with an increased risk, naproxen being the least harmful. [Trelle et al, 2011]. Since 44% of OA patients may be at a high CV risk and a further 28% at moderate risk [Lanas et al, 2010] caution is required when prescribing a NSAID. Therefore, CV risk should be assessed in all patients with OA [Singh et al, 2002; Kadam et al, 2004; Stürmer et al, 1998; Marks et al, 2002], and a CV risk stratification is highly recommended before NSAID prescription. CV risk can be estimated by either the Framingham 10-year risk score for CV events [Wilson et al, 1998] or the SCORE project [Conroy et al, 2003]. These risk scores take into account traditional CV risk factors, such as age, gender, diabetes, hypertension, cholesterol and smoking, and patients are stratified according to the 10-year risk for a CV event. A 10-year risk of 20% or more is considered high, and corresponds to the threshold for risk factor interventions. Naproxen plus PPI is preferred for patients with high CV risk, if needed. For patients with high CV and high GI risk, NSAIDs are not recommended [Burmester et al, 2011].

2.2. Special Circumstances

2.2.1. Asthma

Exacerbation of asthma has been reported with salicylate, but can be seen with other NSAIDs as well. COX-2 selective NSAIDs may be safe in patients with aspirin-sensitive asthma but data is limited [West and Fernandez, 2003].

2.2.2. G-6-PD Deficiency

Patients with G-6-PD deficiency should avoid aspirin. Sulfonamide derivatives, such as Celecoxib, should also be avoided in these patients.

2.2.3. Pregnancy and Lactation

Few patients with OA may fall into this category. Non selective NSAIDs are considered safe during the first two trimesters of pregnancy, but they should not be used in the third trimester of pregnancy, because they cause premature closure of ductus arteriosus [Schoenfeld et al, 1992]. Short-term use of non selective NSAIDs (preferably of short half-life) and aspirin are considered compatible with breastfeeding [American Academy of Pediatrics

Committee on drugs Pediatrics, 1989]. Data on the safety of COX-2 selective inhibitors during pregnancy and breastfeeding is limited.

2.3. Topical NSAIDs

Topical NSAIDs have been developed in an attempt to minimize toxicity from systemic NSAIDs. Topical NSAID preparations, such as diclofenac and aceclofenac, have shown symptomatic efficacy superior to placebo [Towheed et al, 2006; Moore et al, 1998] and comparable to oral NSAIDs in knee and hand OA [Tugwell et al, 2004; Moore et al, 1998].

Adverse effects. Systemic exposure from topical NSAIDs is limited, and side effects do not substantially differ from placebo [Moore et al, 1998]. Renal and CV side effects have not been reported, and GI complications are infrequent and do not include ulcer, bleeding or perforation. Common adverse effects of topical preparations include local skin reactions, mostly dry skin, and rash [Barthel et al, 2010].

3. Intra-Articular Corticosteroids

A systematic review of 28 trials, including 1,973 patients, showed efficacy of intra-articular (IA) corticosteroids (CS) for pain over placebo, but this effect was short-lived [Bellamy et al, 2006b]. Triamcinolone hexacetonide was superior to betamethasone. Comparison between IA CS and IA hyaluronic acid (HA) did not show any difference up to 4 weeks post-injection, but IA HA was superior from week 5 to week 13. IA CS did not differ in efficacy from joint lavage [Bellamy et al, 2006b]. The combination of IA CS with joint lavage may have an additive effect [Ravaud et al, 1999], especially in patients with more severe disease [Parmigiani et al, 2010]. Predictors of good response include thorough aspiration of the joint before injection [Gaffney et al, 1995] and absence of inflammation on ultrasound [Chao et al, 2010].

Systemic absorption of CS takes place shortly after IA administration [Gray et al, 1981], but systemic adverse events are uncommon. There may be a temporary increase of blood glucose levels in diabetic patients [Habibet al, 2009], whereas iatrogenic infection occurs very rarely [Gray et al, 1981; Pal and Morris, 1999]. Strict adherence to aseptic technique eliminates the risk of iatrogenic infection.

A point of debate has been the effect of IA CS on cartilage. Biopsies from patients participating in an RCT revealed amelioration of OA lesions [Guidolin et al, 2001] and IA CS knee joint injections every 3 months for up to

2 years did not have deleterious effects on the structure of the joint [Raynauld et al, 2003]. Similarly, IA CS injection did not increase the rate of joint replacement in patients with rheumatoid arthritis (RA) [Roberts et al, 1996]. On the other hand, IA CS plus anaesthetic resulted in increased chondrocyte apoptosis [Farkas et al, 2010] and knees injected with CS showed more radiographic progression than non-injected knees. A selection bias may be operative in non-RCTs, since knees with more severe disease could be eligible for injections [Wada et al, 1993].

4. Intra-Articular Hyaluronic Acid

Hyaluronic acid (HA) is a glucosaminoglycan naturally present in synovial fluid (Lo et al, 2003). Preparations with molecular weight (mw) between 500-7,000 kDa are available, with high mw molecules achieving a longer half-life within the joint. Viscosupplementation with HA showed superior efficacy over placebo and comparable to NSAIDs for pain and function [Bellamy et al, 2006a; Wang et al, 2004], but the size effect is modest [Lo et al, 2003], and of questionable clinical significance [Arrich et al, 2005]. Methodological issues over sample size and heterogeneity of studies make interpretation of results difficult [Bellamy et al, 2006a; Wang et al, 2004; Lo et al, 2003; Arrich et al, 2005].

Indirect comparisons favour high mw HA (hylan) over standard preparations [Lo et al, 2003, Wang et al, 2004], but meta-analyses of direct comparisons found no significant difference between high and standard mw preparations [Reichenbach et al, 2007a] or any difference among different preparations [Bellamy et al, 2006a]. Two large recent RCTs found no difference in the efficacy between high and standard mw HA [Juni et al, 2007; Onel et al, 2008].

Adverse events are uncommon. A post-injection increase in swelling and pain can be seen, more commonly with high than standard mw HA [Reichenbach et al, 2007a].

5. Diacerein

Diacerein has anti-inflammatory properties, inhibiting the production and activity of interleukin (IL)-1β [Martel-Pelletier et al, 1998, Moldovan et al, 2000]. Meta-analyses of RCTs found that diacerein (100mg daily) was more efficacious than placebo for pain and function, and comparable to NSAIDs, [Rintelen et al, 2006, Bartels et al, 2010; Fidelix et al, 2006]. In addition, diacerein showed a carry-over effect for 3 months after treatment discontinuation.

Diacerein may have a structure-modifying potential. Treatment of hip OA for 3 years had a significant structure-modifying effect compared to placebo [Dougados et al, 2001], but treatment of knee OA for one year did not retard radiographic progression [Pham et al, 2004].

The most frequent side effect of diacerein is diarrhea (25%) followed by abdominal pain [Bartels et al, 2010] and is the main reason for treatment discontinuation (up to 18%) [Fidelix et al, 2006]. Diacerein can be used in patients intolerant or with contraindications to NSAIDs [Bartels et al, 2010].

6. Glucozamine and Chondroitin Sulfate

Both glucozamine and chondroitin sulphate are normal constituents of human cartilage. They are used in OA but their efficacy is questionable. Early meta-analyses found that glucosamine and chondroitin are efficacious for symptom relief and function improvement [McAlindon et al, 2000, Towheed et al, 2005, Richy et al, 2003, Leeb et al, 2000], but recent meta-analyses showed that the symptomatic benefit of chondroitin [Reichenbach et al, 2007b], glucosamine [Vlad et al, 2007], and their combination [Wandel et al, 2010] is none to minimal, probably because of a large RCT with negative results [Clegg et al, 2006]. This latter RCT, however, did show a symptomatic efficacy of the chondroitin and glucosamine hydrochloride combination in patients with moderate-to-severe pain [Clegg et al, 2006]. Glucosamine sulphate appears to be somewhat more efficacious than glucosamine hydrochloride [Wandel et al, 2010, Towheed et al, 2005, Vlad et al, 2007]. However, the size effect is small and heterogeneity between studies considerable, thus making the clinical significance of the results questionable [Wandel et al, 2010]. Glucozamine sulphate may have structure-modifying properties in knee OA. RCTs and meta-analyses in knee OA showed a small but significant slowing of joint space loss [Reginster at al, 2001, Pavelka et al, 2002; Towheed et al, 2005, Richy et al, 2003, Poolsup et al, 2005]. Furthermore, patients on glucosamine sulfate had fewer joint replacement surgeries at 5 years [Bruyere et al, 2008]. A RCT of glucosamine sulphate in hip OA did not show any protective effect [Rozendaal et al, 2008]. Glucozamine hydrochloride failed to show any structure protective effect [Clegg et al, 2006]. The potential of chondroitin to slow radiographic progression is supported by four meta-analyses of RCTs [Bana et al, 2006, Reichenbach et al, 2007b, Hochberg et al, 2008, Hochberg, 2010]. However, the size effect is small and not universally accompanied by symptomatic relief, raising questions for its clinical significance [Bana et al, 2006, Reichenbach et al, 2007b]. A recent meta-analysis [Wandel et al, 2010) and a large RCT [Clegg et al, 2006] failed to show a joint protective effect of chondroitin. A RCT in knee OA using MRI found that chondroitin reduces cartilage volume loss at 6 and 12 months [Wildi et al, 2011]. Chondroitin sulfate also reduced bone marrow lesions, which are associated with cartilage loss and progressive joint destruction in OA [Felson et al, 2003, Tanamas et al, 2010, Davies-Tuck et al, 2010, Dore et al, 2010].

Glucozamine and chondroitin are not associated with any significant adverse effects [Towheed et al., 2005].

7. Other Drugs

7.1. Bone Antiresorptive Agents

Bone antiresorptive agents, such as for biphosphonates, calcitonin and estrogens, that are used for osteoporosis, showed chondroprotective effects in animal models of OA [Hayami et al, 2004, Sondergaard et al, 2007]. Biphosphonates have been associated with less pronounced bone marrow lesions and pain in knee OA [Carbone et al, 2004]. However, a 2-year RCT of risendronate failed to relieve symptoms or to slow radiographic progression of knee OA [Bingham et al, 2006]. Another RCT found significant improvements only in patient's global assessment and use of walking aids in the 15 mg/day group, with no significant effect on structure [Spector et al, 2005]. A randomized, phase II trial comparing IA clodronate with IA HA injections in knee OA found similar improvements for pain [Rossini et al, 2009].

Alendronate and strondium renalate were found to retard spinal osteophytes [Neogi et al, 2008] and disk-space narrowing progression [Neogi et al, 2008, Bryere et al, 2008] in patients with osteoporosis and spinal OA. A formulation of salmon calcitonin for oral use showed improvement in function and reduction of biochemical biomarkers of cartilage degradation in a small RCT [Manicourt et al, 2006].

Despite the chondroprotective potential of biphosphonates, calcitonin or strontium ranelate, both symptom and structure-modifying effect have not been proved, and further studies are needed.

7.2. Rheumatoid Arthritis Disease Modifying Drugs in OA

There is growing evidence that synovial inflammation contributes to symptoms and signs of OA. It is therefore anticipated that inhibition of the inflammatory component of OA may provide effective therapeutic intervention for this disease.

7.2.1. Methotrexate

Methotrexate (MTX) showed limited efficacy in experimental models of OA [Neidel et al. 1998]. In a lapine partial medial meniscectomy model of OA, MTX failed to affect metalloproteinase (MMP) and tissue inhibitors of metalloproteinase levels in articular cartilage [Mannoni et al, 1993].

A conjugate of MTX with HA for IA injection, designed to deliver two agents but minimize the risks of MTX, significantly reduced knee swelling in rats with antigen-induced arthritis [Homma et al, 2009].

A Phase III, RCT comparing methotrexate 10 mg/week with placebo for one year in erosive hand OA is ongoing [NCT01068405].

7.2.2. Hydroxychloroquine

In vitro, hydroxychloroquine (HCQ) was found to suppress IL-1β-induced NO production in human OA cartilage, indicating a potential therapeutic value in OA [Vuolteenaho et al, 2005]. However, in vivo, only retrospective studies with very small number of patients are available. HCQ was efficacious in 6 of the 8 patients with erosive OA unresponsive to NSAIDs [Bryant et al, 1995]. Punzi et al allocated 15 patients with erosive OA to receive HCQ or traditional analgesic or NSAIDs for one year; significant improvements in ESR and soluble IL-2 receptor at 12 months and in the Ritchie index at 6 and 12 months were seen in patients treated with HCQ [Punzi et al, 1996]. HCQ seems also to be efficacious in OA associated with calcium-containing crystals [Wu et al, 2005]. A prospective RCT is ongoing in the Netherlands [NCT01148043], while a randomized, single blind study will evaluate the efficacy and safety of prednisolone and chloroquine add-on therapy in knee OA patients treated with a combination of glucosamine and chondroitin sulfate [NCT00805519].

7.3. Biologics in OA

7.3.1. IL-1RA

IL-1 blockade with IL-1 receptor antagonist (IL-1RA) can slow down progression of disease in animal models of OA [Caron et al, 1996; Pelletier et al 1997; Fernandes et al 1999]. Anakinra (IL-1RA) (100 mg/day, SC) was tried in 3 women with severe EOA unresponsive to conventional therapy. After 3 months, there was an improvement in pain, and global assessment, whereas NSAIDs were withdrawn [Bacconnier et al, ARD 2009]. IA injection of Anakinra in knee OA was safe [Chevalier et al, 2005, Chevalier et al, 2009] but ineffective [Chevalier et al, 2009].

A trial of intra-articular canakinumab, an anti-IL-1 monoclonal antibody, in knee OA is ongoing [NCT01160822].

7.3.2. TNFα Inhibitors

In an open-label pilot trial in 12 patients with erosive OA, adalimumab (human anti-TNFα monoclonal antibody) (40 mg/2weeks) for 12 weeks significantly improved the number of swollen joints and improved modestly all efficacy measures [Magnano et al, 2007]. A pilot study of intra-articular injections of infliximab (chimeric anti-TNFα monoclonal antibody) in interphalangeal joints of hands (0.2 mL [0.1 mg/mL] in each affected joint) of 10 women with erosive OA showed relief from pain at 6 months and reduction of radiographic progression at 12 months, without local or systemic adverse reactions. [Fioravanti et al, 2009]

Adalimumab will be tested in a RCT, phase III, in severe hand OA, unresponsive to NSAIDs and analgesics [NCT00597623], and an open-label study in knee OA [NCT00686439]. Another study will determine if infliximab will reduce inflammation in the synovial membrane in early knee OA [NCT01144143]

8. New Drugs

8.1. COX-Inhibiting Nitric Oxide Donators (CINODs)

COX-inhibiting nitric oxide donators (CINODs) are a new class of anti-inflammatory drugs designed to combine the anti-inflammatory effects of the parent COX inhibitor with vasodilating effects of nitric oxide (NO) to improve the GI and CV safety profile of the parent NSAID [Wallace et al, 2009]. NO derived from CINODs increases gastric mucosal blood flow, inhibits leukocyte adhesion to GI microcirculation, increases mucus secretion and bicarbonate secretion, and facilitates epithelial repair [Wallace et al, 1994a; Wallace et al, 1994c; Fiorucci et al, 1999]. These favorable effects counteract the detrimental effects of parent NSAID on gastric mucosa [Elliott et al, 1995; Brzozowska et al, 2004]. NO derived from CINODs exerts cardioprotective effects, by increasing vasodilatation, and inhibiting platelet aggregation [Wallace et al, 1995; Momi et al, 2000]. It can also have anti-inflammatory properties, since it inhibits Nuclear Factor kappa-B (NFkB) [Wallace et al, 2009].

The first member of the CINOD class is naproxcinod. In pre-clinical studies, naproxcinod was as effective as the parent naproxen in reducing pain and swelling in several animal models, but with less GI hemorrhagic damage [Davies et al, 1997; Cicala et al, 2000; Ellis et al, 2005]. In addition, coadministration of naproxcinod with aspirin in rat arthritic models did not exacerbate gastric mucosal injury caused by aspirin [Fiorucci et al, 2004]. Naproxcinod had a blood pressure lowering effect in several animal models of hypertension [Muscara et al, 1998; Muscara et al, 2000; Muscara et al, 2001; Presotto et al, 2006], while it did not affect blood pressure in normotensive rats [Muscara et al, 2000; Presotto et al, 2006]. In a model of acute ischemia and reperfusion of the rabbit heart, naproxcinod showed significant anti-ischemic properties [Rossoni et al, 2004]. The cardioprotective properties of naproxcinod were confirmed in vivo in rats [Rossoni et al, 2006].

The efficacy of naproxcinod (750 mg bid which is equipotent to naproxen 500 mg bid) showed similar efficacy to naproxen in hip and knee OA in RCTs [Baerwald et al, 2010; Karlsson et al, 2009; Lohmander et al, 2005; Schnitzer et al, 2005; Schnitzer et al, 2010; Schnitzer et al, 2011]. Naproxcinod also had a better GI and CV safety profile than naproxen. Naproxcinod 750mg bid showed fewer endoscopic erosions than naproxen 500 mg bid in healthy volunteers at 12 days [Hawkey et al, 2003] but this difference did not reach statistical significance in OA patients at 6 weeks (Lohmander et al, 2005). Naproxcinod (750 mg bid) did not change blood pressure in hip and knee OA patients participating in RCTs [White et al, 2011]. In these patients naproxen increased blood pressure, particularly in hypertensive patients treated with renin-angiotensin blockers or diuretics [White et al, 2011; White et al, 2009]. There was no rebound effect on blood pressure after discontinuation of naproxcinod. Postural hypotension was slightly more frequently in the naproxcinod group, but infrequently led to discontinuation of treatment [Schnitzer et al, 2011].

Naproxcinod most probably will find a place in patients with increased CV and GI risk.

8.2. COX/LOX Inhibitors

The inhibition of COX with traditional NSAIDs may enforce the alternative pathway of arachidonic acid, namely the 5-lipo-oxygenase (5-LOX) pathway with production of more leukotrienes [Parades et al, 2002; Marcouiller et al, 2005; Martel-Pelletier et al, 2003]. Leukotrienes are pro-inflammatory molecules and cause gastric damage. They are chemotactic for leukocytes, increase pro-inflammatory cytokines, induce vasoconstriction in gastric mucosa, and stimulate secretion of gastric acid [Rainsford et al, 1996; Jovanovic et al, 2001; He et al, 2002; Fiorucci et al, 2001]. They also stimulate bone resorption and cause bronchoconstriction [Abraham et al, 1997; Pelletier et al, 2004]. The pro-inflammatory actions of leukotrienes have led to the concept that NSAIDs may accelerate the progression of OA [Huskisson et al, 1995]. This has led to the development of dual COX/5-LOX inhibitors to have better anti-inflammatory and safety profile than traditional NSAIDs [Fiorucci et al, 2001].

Several chemically different COX/5-LOX inhibitors have been used in preclinical or clinical studies, with licofelone being the first one to be tested in RCTs [Reginster et al, 2002].

Licofelone has anti-inflammatory, analgesic, antipyretic and anti-platelet activities [Singh et al, 2006]. It reduced synovial cell proliferation and bone and cartilage erosions in an adjuvant arthritis model [Gay et al, 2001]. It also reduced the development of structural damage in an OA animal model [Jovanovic et al, 2001].

Licofelone was as effective as naproxen and celecoxib in knee OA in RCTs [Reginster et al, 2002; Pavelka et al, 2003; Blanco et al, 2003]. Furthermore, licofelone significantly reduced cartilage loss in knee OA [Raynauld et al, 2009].

Licofelone has a lower ulcerogenic potential than aspirin, indomethacin and diclofenac [Wallace et al 1994b]. In an endoscopic study of 121 volunteers randomly assigned to a 4-week treatment with licofelone 200 mg twice daily (bid) or 400 mg bid, placebo or naproxen 500 mg bid, ulcers were observed in 20% of the naproxen group and none in the licofelone and placebo groups [Buchner et al 2003; Klesser et al 2004]. In addition, it does not exacerbate gastric mucosal damage, even in aspirin-treated rats [Fiorrucci

2003], an observation confirmed also in human beings [Buchner 2003]. Licofelone had better tolerability, including peripheral oedema and hypertension, compared to celecoxib and naproxen in RCTs [Reginster et al 2002; Pavelka et al 2003; Blanco et al 2003].

8.3. Apremilast

Apremilast is an oral type 4 phosphodiesterase (PDE4) inhibitor. Inhibition of PDE4 has previously been shown to suppress immune and inflammatory responses [Sekut et al 1995; Schafer et al 2010]. It reduces TNFα production from synovial cells of RA patients and significantly suppresses experimental arthritis [McCann et al. 2010]. There is an ongoing RCT of apremilast 20 mg bid for erosive OA [NCT01200472].

8.4. Icatibant

Icatibant is a selective bradykinin B2 receptor antagonist. Bradykinins (BKs) are key mediators of pain in knee OA and act directly by activation of BK2 receptors and indirectly by increasing the release of prostaglandins, cytokines and histamine [Blais et al 1997; Tonussi et al 1997; Sharma et al 1996; Marceau et al 2004]. BK and leukotriene B4 concentrations in synovial fluid were found to correlate with the severity of synovitis [Nishimura et al 2002]. Icatibant, a synthetic decapeptide [Rhaleb et al 1992], showed efficacy in vitro [Regoli et al 1998] and in vivo models of inflammation [Perkins et al 1993; Davis et al 1994; Levy et al 2000; Damas et al 1992]. It showed a significant analgesic effect in knee OA in a RCT, but failed to show a significant anti-inflammatory efficacy [Song et al 2009]. The analgesic effect of icatibant can be partly explained by inhibition of nociceptive neurons [Regoli et al 1998].

8.5. Matrix Metelloproteinases (MMPs) Inhibitors

Matrix metalloproteinases (MMPs) are a group of proteolytic enzymes that degrade cartilage extracellular matrix. MMPs have been implicated in joint destruction that occurs in arthritis, and MMP inhibitors have been thought of as good therapeutic targets in RA and OA. Despite promising data in animal models [Fujisawa et al 2002; Lewis et al 1997; Brewster et al 1998; Close DR 2001], studies in humans did not progress for safety issues revealed in cancer studies [Hirte et al 2006]. A study in OA confirmed that a PG-116800 MMP inhibitor is unsuitable for OA [Krzeski et al 2007].

8.6. Botulinum Toxin Type A

Botulinum (BoNT) toxin, apart for its muscle paralyzing effects used for the treatment of cervical dystonia and blephrospasm, has anti-nociceptive properties [Singh JA 2010]. A single IA BoTNA (100 units) into glenohumeral OA or RA joint refractory to IA corticosteroids and oral medications resulted in pain improvement. [Singh et al. 2009]. A single IA BoTNA injection was also efficacious in pain improvement in knee OA [Boon et al 2010; Chou et al 2010] and in total knee replacement [Singh JA 2010]. Injection of BoNT-A into the adductor muscles reduced pain and improved mobility and quality of life in patients hip OA [Marchini et al. 2010]. These studies support the option of BoNT-A as a pain relief medication in knee OA.

8.7. Antibiotics

8.7.1. Tetracyclines

Tetracyclines can inhibit MMPs and prevent tissue destruction independent of their antimicrobial activity. However, a pilot study of doxycycline for advanced OA of temporomandibular joint (TMJ) [Israel et al 1998] and a RCT trial for knee OA [Mazzuca et al 2004] failed to show symptomatic improvement. The small retardation of joint space narrowing was of questionable clinical value and outweighed by safety problems [Brandt et al, 2005; Nüesch et al 2009c].

8.7.2. Macrolides

Erythromycin in a RCT of knee OA improved joint effusion, pain, and joint function [Sadreddini et al 2009].

CONCLUSION

OA treatment thus far is far from satisfactory. The first therapeutic intervention in OA is traditional analgesics. In patients with moderate to severe pain, NSAIDs or selective COX-2 inhibitors can be prescribed. However, cardiovascular and gastrointestinal safety issues have led to novel drugs, such as cyclo-oxygenase-inhibiting, nitric oxide donor drugs (naproxcinod) and dual cyclo-oxygenase and 5-lipoxygenase inhibitors (licofelone). The goal of disease modification is to be proved, and new trials using MRI as end points are expected to help. Therapeutic interventions targeting inflammation, bone metabolism, mediators of pain are under study.

REFERENCES

Abadie E, Ethgen D, Avouac B, Bouvenot G, Branco J, Bruyere O, Calvo G, Devogelaer JP, Dreiser RL, Herrero-Beaumont G, Kahan A, Kreutz G, Laslop A, Lemmel EM, Nuki G, Van De Putte L, Vanhaelst L, Reginster JY; Group for the Respect of Excellence and Ethics in Science. Recommendations for the use of new methods to assess the efficacy of disease-modifying drugs in the treatment of osteoarthritis. *Osteoarthritis Cartilage* 2004;12:263-8.

Abraham WM, Laufer S, Tries S. The effects of ML3000 on antigen induced responses in sheep. *Pulm Pharmacol. Ther.* 1997;10:167–73.

American Academy of Pediatrics: Committee on drugs. The transfer of drugs and other chemicals into human milk. *Pediatrics* 2001;108:776-789.

Amin S, LaValley MP, Guermazi A, Grigoryan M, Hunter DJ, Clancy M, Niu J, Gale DR, Felson DT. The relationship between cartilage loss on magnetic resonance imaging and radiographic progression in men and women with knee osteoarthritis. *Arthritis Rheum* 2005;52:3152-9.

Arrich J, Piribauer F, Mad P, Schmid D, Klaushofer K, Mullner M. Intra-articular hyaluronic acid for the treatment of osteoarthritis of the knee: systematic review and meta-analysis. *CMAJ* 2005;172. DOI:10.1503/cmaj.1041203.

Ayral X, Pickering EH, Woodworth TG, Mackillop N, Dougados M. Synovitis: a potential predictive factor of structural progression of medial tibiofemoral knee osteoarthritis -- results of a 1 year longitudinal arthroscopic study in 422 patients. *Osteoarthritis Cartilage* 2005;13:361-7.

Bacconnier L, Jorgensen C, Fabre S. Erosive osteoarthritis of the hand: clinical experience with anakinra. *Ann. Rheum. Dis.* 2009; 68: 1078-9.

Baerwald C, Verdecchia P, Duquesroix B, Frayssinet H, Ferreira T. Efficacy, safety, and effects on blood pressure of naproxcinod 750 mg twice daily compared with placebo and naproxen 500 mg twice daily in patients with osteoarthritis of the hip: a randomized, double-blind, parallel-group, multicenter study. *Arthritis Rheum* 2010;62:3635-44.

Bannwarth B, Gastrointestinal safety of paracetamol: is there any cause for concern? *Expert Opin. Drug Saf* 2004;3:269-72.

Bartels EM, Bliddal H, Schøndorff PK, Altman RD, Zhang W, Christensen R. Symptomatic efficacy and safety of diacerein in the treatment of osteoarthritis: a meta-analysis of randomized placebo-controlled trials. *Osteoarthritis Cartilage* 2010;18:289-96.

Barthel HR, Axford-Gatley RA, Topical nonsteroidal anti-inflammatory drugs for osteoarthritis. *Postgrad Med.* 2010;122:98-106.

Batlle-Gualda E, Román Ivorra J, Martín-Mola E, Carbonell Abelló J, Linares Ferrando LF, Tornero Molina J, Raber Béjar A, Fortea Busquets J.Aceclofenac vs paracetamol in the management of symptomatic osteoarthritis of the knee: a double-blind 6-week randomized controlled trial. *Osteoarthritis Cartilage* 2007;15:900-8.

Beaulieu AD, Peloso PM, Haraoui B, Bensen W, Thomson G, Wade J, Quigley P, Eisenhoffer J, Harsanyi Z, Darke AC. Once-daily, controlled-release tramadol and sustained-release diclofenac relieve chronic pain due to osteoarthritis: a randomized controlled trial. *Pain Res Manage* 2008;13:103-10.

Bellamy N, Campbell J, Welch V, Gee TL, Bourne R, Wells GA. Viscosupplementation for the treatment of osteoarthritis of the knee. *Cochrane Database Syst Rev.* 2006a;(2): CD005321.

Bellamy N, Campbell J,Welch V, Gee TL, Bourne R, Wells GA. Intraarticular corticosteroid for treatment of osteoarthritis of the knee. *Cochrane Database Syst Rev* 2006b;(2): CD005328.

Blais C Jr, Couture R, Drapeau G, Colman RW, Adam A. Involvement of endogenous kinins in the pathogenesis of peptidoglycan-induced arthritis in the Lewis rat. *Arthritis Rheum* 1997;40:1327–33.

Blanco F, Buchner A, Bias P, et al. Licofelone, an inhibitor of COX-1, COX-2 and 5-LOX, is as effective as naproxen and shows improved safety during 12 months of treatment in patients with osteoarthritis of the knee [abstract]. *Ann. Rheum Dis*, 2003;62(Suppl. 1):262, FRI0217.

Boon AJ, Smith J, Dahm DL, Sorenson EJ, Larson DR, Fitz-Gibbon PD, Dykstra DD, Singh JA Efficacy of intra-articular botulinum toxin type A in painful knee osteoarthritis: a pilot study. *PMR* 2010; 2(4): 268-76.

Brandt KD, Mazzuca SA, Katz BP, Lane KA, Buckwalter KA, Yocum DE, Wolfe F, Schnitzer TJ, Moreland LW, Manzi S, Bradley JD, Sharma L, Oddis CV, Hugenberg ST, Heck LW. Effects of doxycycline on progression of osteoarthritis. Results of a randomized, placebo-controlled double-blind trial. *Arthritis Rheum* 2005;52:2015-25.

Brater DC, Harris C, Redfern JS, Gertz BJ. Renal effects of COX-2-selective inhibitors. *Am. J. Nephrol* 2001;21:1-15.

Brewster M, Lewis EJ, Wilson KL, Greenham AK, Bottomley KM. Ro 32-3555, an orally active collagenase selective inhibitor, prevents structural damage in the STR/ORT mouse model of osteoarthritis. *Arthritis Rheum* 1998; 41:1639-44.

Brooks P. Non-steroidal anti-inflammatory drugs. Oxford Textbook of Rheumatology, 2nd ed, 1998, Oxford University Press. Eds Maddison PJ, Isenberg DA, Woo P, Glass DN, pp575-581.

Brooks PM, Day RO. Nonsteroidal antiinflammatory drugs – differences and similarities. *N Engl. J. Med.* 1991;324:1716-25.

Brown TJ, Hooper L, Elliott RA, Payne K, Webb R, Roberts C, Rostom A, Symmons D. A comparison of the cost-effectiveness of five strategies for the prevention of non-steroidal anti-inflammatory drug-induced gastrointestinal toxicity: a systematic review with economic modelling. *Health Technol Assess* 2006;10(38).

Bryant LR, des Rosier KF, Carpenter MT. Hydroxychloroquine in the treatment of erosive osteoarthritis. *J. Rheumatol.* 1995; 22: 1527-31.

Brzozowska I. Targosz A, Sliwowski Z, Kwiecien S, Drozdowicz D, Pajdo R, Konturek PC, Brzozowski T, Pawlik M, Konturek SJ, Pawlik WW, Hahn EG.. Healing of chronic gastric ulcers in diabetic rats treated with native aspirin, nitric oxide (NO)-derivative of aspirin and cyclooxygenase (COX)-2 inhibitor. *J. Physiol. Pharmacol.* 2004;55: 773– 90.

Buchner A, Bias P, Lammerich A. Twice the therapeutic dose of licofelone–an inhibitor of COX-1, COX-2 and 5-LOX–results in a significantly lower gastrointestinal ulcer incidence than naproxen in osteoarthritis patients, when administered with or without concomitant low-dose aspirin. *Ann. Rheum Dis*, 2003;62(1 Suppl.):261.

Buckwalter JA, Saltzman C, Brown T. The impact of osteoarthritis: implications for research. *Clin. Orthop Relat Res.* 2004;427(Suppl):S6-S15.

Burmester G, Lanas A, Biasucci A, Hermann M, Lohmander S, Olivieri I, Scarpignato C, Smolen J, Hawkey C, Bajkowski A, Berenbaum F, Breedveld F, Dieleman P, Dougados M, MacDonald T, Martin Mola E, Mets T, Van Den Noortgate N, Stoevelaar H. The appropriate use of non-steroidal antiinflammatory drugs in rheumatic disease: opinions of a multidisciplinary European expert panel. *Ann. Rheum. Dis.* 2011 (e-pub ahead of print). doi:10.1136/ard.2010.128660.

Caron JP, Fernandes JC, Martel-Pelletier J, Tardif G, Mineau F, Geng C, Pelletier JP. Chondroprotective effect of intraarticular injections of interleukin-1 receptor antagonist in experimental osteoarthritis: suppression of collagenase-1 expression. *Arthritis Rheum* 1996;39:1535–44.

Cepeda MS, Camargo F, Zea C, Valencia L. Tramadol for osteoarthritis: a systematic review and metaanalysis. *J. Rheumatol.* 2007;34:543-55.

Cepeda MS, Camargo F, Zea C, Valencia L. Tramadol for osteoarthritis. *Cochrane Database Syst Rev* 2006;(3): CD005522.

Chao J, Wu C, Sun B, Hose MK, Quan A, Hughes TH, Boyle D, Kalunian KC. Inflammatory characteristics on ultrasound predict poorer longterm response to intraarticular corticosteroid injections in knee osteoarthritis. *J. Rheumatol* 2010;37:650-5.

Chevalier X, Giraudeau B, Conrozier T, Marliere J, Kiefer P, Goupille P. safety study of intraarticular injection of interleukin 1 receptor antagonist in patients with painful knee osteoarthritis: a multicenter study. *J. Rheumatol.* 2005; 32: 1317-23.

Chevalier X, Goupille P, Beaulieu AD, Burch FX, Bensen WG, Conrozier T, Loeuille D, Kivitz AJ, Silver D, Appleton BE. Intraarticular injection of anakinra in osteoarthritis of the knee: a multicenter, randomized, double-blind, placebo-controlled study. *Arthritis Rheum.* 2009;61:344-52.

Chou CL, Lee SH, Lu SY, Tsai KL, Ho CY, Lai HC. Therapeutic effects of intra-articular botulinum neurotoxin in advanced knee osteoarthritis. J *Clin. Med. Assoc.* 2010; 73(11): 573-80.

Chou R HM, Peterson K, Dana T, Roberts C. Comparative Effectiveness and Safety of Analgesics for Osteoarthritis. Comparative Effectiveness Review No. 4. Rockville, MD: *Agency for Healthcare Research and Quality;* 2006.

Cicala C, Ianaro A, Fiorucci S, Calignano A, Bucci M, Gerli R, Santucci L, Wallace JL, Cirino G. NO-naproxen modulates inflammation, nociception and downregulates T cell response in rat Freund's adjuvant arthritis. *Br. J. Pharmacol.* 2000; 130: 1399–405.

Clegg DO, Reda DJ, Harris CL, Klein MA, O'Dell JR, Hooper MM, Bradley JD, Bingham CO 3rd, Weisman MH, Jackson CG, Lane NE, Cush JJ, Moreland LW, Schumacher HR Jr, Oddis CV, Wolfe F, Molitor JA, Yocum DE, Schnitzer TJ, Furst DE, Sawitzke AD, Shi H, Brandt KD, Moskowitz RW, Williams HJ. Glucosamine, chondroitin sulfate, and the two in combination for painful knee osteoarthritis. *N. Engl. J. Med.* 2006;354:795-808.

Close DR. Matrix metalloproteinase inhibitors in rheumatic diseases. *Ann. Rheum. Dis.* 2001; 60(Suppl 3):iii62-67.

Conroy RM, Pyorala K, Fitzgerald AP, Sans S, Menotti A, De Backer G, Ducimetiere P, Jousilahti P, Keil U, Njolstad I, Oganov RG, Thomsen T, Tunstall-Pedoe H, Tverdal A, Wedel H, Whincup P, Wilhemsen L, Graham IM, on behalf of the SCORE project group. Estimation of the ten-year risk of fatal cardiovascular disease in Europe: the SCORE project. *Eur. Heart J.* 2003;24:987-1003.

Damas J, Remacle-Volon G. Influence of a long-acting bradykinin antagonist, Hoe 140, on some acute inflammatory reactions in the rat. *Eur. J. Pharmacol* 1992;211:81–86.

Davies NM, Roseth AG, Appleyard CB, McKnight W, Del Soldato P, Calignano A, Cirino G, Wallace JL. NO-naproxen vs. naproxen: ulcerogenic, analgesic and anti-inflammatory effects. *Aliment. Pharmacol. Ther.* 1997;11: 69–79.

Davis AJ, Perkins MN. The involvement of bradykinin B1 and B2 receptor mechanisms in cytokine-induced mechanical hyperalgesia in the rat. *Br. J. Pharmacol.* 1994;113:63–8.

Dougados M, Nguyen M, Berdah L, Maziéres B, Vignon E, Lequesne M; ECHODIAH Investigators Study Group. Evaluation of the structure-modifying effects of diacerein in hip osteoarthritis: ECHODIAH, a three-year, placebo-controlled trial. Evaluation of the Chondromodulating Effect of Diacerein in OA of the Hip. *Arthritis Rheum* 2001;44:2539-47.

Elliott SN, McKnight W, Cirino G, Wallace JL. A nitric oxide-releasing nonsteroidal anti-inflammatory drug accelerates gastric ulcer healing in rats. *Gastroenterology* 1995;109: 524–30.

Ellis JL, Augustyniak ME, Cochran ED, Earl RA, Garvey DS, Gordon LJ, Janero DR, Khanapure SP, Letts LG, Melim TL, Murty MG, Schwalb DJ, Shumway MJ, Selig WM, Trocha AM, Young DV, Zemtseva IS. NMI-1182, a gastro-protective cyclo-oxygenase inhibiting nitric oxide donor. *Inflammopharmacology* 2005;12: 521–34.

Farkas B, Kvell K, Czömpöly T, Illés T, Bárdos T. Increased chondrocyte death after steroid and local anesthetic combination. *Clin. Orthop Relat Res.* 2010;468:3112-20.

Fernandes J, Tardif G, Martel-Pelletier J, Lascau-Coman V, Dupuis M, Moldovan F, Sheppard M, Krishnan BR, Pelletier JP. In vivo transfer of interleukin-1 receptor antagonist gene in osteoarthritic rabbit knee joints: prevention of osteoarthritis progression. *Am. J. Pathol.* 1999; 154:1159–69.

Fidelix TS, Soares B, FernandesMoça Trevisani V. Diacerein for osteoarthritis. *Cochrane Database Syst Rev* 2006;(1): CD005117.

Fioravanti A, Fabbroni M, Cerase A, Galeazzi M. Treatment of erosive osteoarthritis of the hands by intraarticular infliximab injections: a pilot study. *Rheumatol Int* 2009; 29: 961-5.

Fiorucci S, Di Lorenzo A, Renga B, Farneti S, Morelli A, Cirino G. Nitric oxide (NO)-releasing naproxen (HCT- 3012 [(S)-6-methoxy-a-methyl-2-naphthaleneacetic acid 4-(nitrooxy)butyl ester]) interactions with aspirin in gastric mucosa of arthritic rats reveal a role for aspirin-triggered lipoxin, prostaglandins, and NO in gastric protection. *J. Pharmacol. Exp. Ther.* 2004;311: 1264–1271.

Fiorucci S, Distrutti E, de Lima OM, Romano M, Mencarelli A, Barbanti M, Palazzini E, Morelli A, Wallace JL. Relative contribution of acetylated cyclo-oxygenase (COX)-2 and 5-lipooxygenase (LOX) in regulating gastric mucosal integrity and adaptation to aspirin. FASEB J, 2003;17(9):1171–1173.

Fiorucci S, Meli R, Bucci M, Cirino G. Dual inhibitors of cyclooxygenase and 5-lipoxygenase. A new avenue in anti-inflammatory therapy? *Biochem. Pharmacol.* 2001; 62: 1433-1438.

Fiorucci S, Santucci L, Federici B, Antonelli E, Distrutti E, Morelli O, Renzo GD, Coata G, Cirino G, Soldato PD, Morelli A. Nitric oxide-releasing NSAIDs inhibit interleukin-1b converting enzyme-like cysteine proteases and protect endothelial cells from apoptosis induced by TNFa. *Aliment. Pharmacol. Ther.* 1999;13: 421–35.

Fishbain DA, Cole B, Lewis J, Rosomoff HL, Rosomoff RS. What percentage of chronic nonmalignant pain patients exposed to chronic opioid analgesic therapy develop abuse/addiction and/or aberrant drug-related behaviors? A structured evidence-based review. *Pain Med.* 2008;9:444-59.

FitzGerald GA, Patrono C. The coxibs, selective inhibitors of cyclooxygenase-2. *N Engl. J. Med.* 2001;345:433-42.

Fransen M, Neal B. Non-steroidal anti-inflammatory drugs for preventing heterotopic bone formation after hip arthroplasty. *Cochrane Database Syst Rev.* 2006;(2):CD001160.

Fujisawa T, Igeta K, Odake S, Morita Y, Yasuda J, Morikawa T. Highly water-soluble matrix metalloproteinases inhibitors and their effects in a rat adjuvant-induced arthritis model. *Bioorg. Med. Chem.* 2002; 10:2569-81.

Gaffney K, Ledingham J, Perry JD Intra-articular triamcinolone hexacetonide in knee osteoarthritis: factors influencing the clinical response. *Ann. Rheum. Dis.* 1995;54:379-81

Garcia Rodriguez LA, Hernández-Díaz S. Relative risk of upper gastrointestinal complications among users of acetaminophen and nonsteroidal anti-inflammatory drugs. *Epidemiology* 2001;12:570-6.

Gardner JS, Blough D, Drinkard CR, Shatin D, Anderson G, Graham D, Alderfer R. Tramadol and seizures: a surveillance study in a managed care population. *Pharmacotherapy* 2000;20:1423-31

Gasse C, Derby L, Vasilakis-Scaramozza C, Jick H. Incid ence of first-time idiopathic seizures in users of tramadol. *Pharmacotherapy* 2000;20:629-34.

Gay RE, Neidhart M, Pataky F, Tries S, Laufer S, Gay S.. Dual inhibition of 5-lipoxygenase and cyclooxygenase 1 and 2 by ML3000 reduces joint destruction in adjuvant arthritis. *J. Rheumatol*, 2001;28:2060–5.

Gray RG, Tenenbaum J, Gottlieb NL. Local corticosteroid injection treatment in rheumatic disorders. *Semin Arthritis Rheum.* 1981;10:231-54

Guccione AA, Felson DT, Anderson JJ, Anthony JM, Zhang Y, Wilson PW, Kelly-Hayes M, Wolf PA, Kreger BE, Kannel WB The effects of specific medical conditions on the functional limitations of elders in the Framingham Study. *Am. J. Public. Health* 1994;84:351–8.

Guidolin DD, Ronchetti IP, Lini E, Guerra D, Frizziero L., Morphological analysis of articular cartilage biopsies from a randomized, clinical study comparing the effects of 500-730 kDa sodium hyaluronate (Hyalgan) and methylprednisolone acetate on primary osteoarthritis of the knee. *Osteoarthritis Cartilage* 2001;9:371-81.

Habib GS. Systemic effects of intra-articular corticosteroids. *Clin. Rheumatol.* 2009;28:749-56.

Hawkey CJ, Jones JI, Atherton CT, Skelly MM, Bebb JR, Fagerholm U, Jonzon B, Karlsson P, Bjarnason IT.. Gastrointestinal safety of AZD3582, a cyclooxygenase inhibiting nitric oxide donator: proof of concept study in humans. *Gut* 2003;52: 1537–42.

He W, Pelletier JP, Martel-Pelletier J, Laufer S, Di Battista JA. Synthesis of interleukin-1beta, tumour necrosis factor-a and interstitial collagenase (MMP-1) is eicosanoid dependent in human OA synovial membrane explants: Interactions with anti-inflammatory cytokines. *J. Rheumatol,* 2002;29:546–53.

Hernandez-Diaz S, Garcia Rodriguez LA. Epidemiologic assessment of the safety of conventional nonsteroidal anti-inflammatory drugs, *Am. J. Med.* 2001; 110(Suppl 3A):20S-27S.

Hirte H, Vergote IB, Jeffrey JR, Grimshaw RN, Coppieters S, Schwartz B, Tu D, Sadura A, Brundage M, Seymour L. A phase III randomized trial of

BAY 12-9566 (tanomastat) as maintenance therapy in patients with advanced ovarian cancer responsive to primary surgery and paclitaxel/platinum containing chemotherapy: a National Cancer Institute of Canada Clinical Trials Group Study. *Gynecol. Oncol.* 2006; 102:300-8.

Homma A, Sato H, Okamachi A, Emura T, Ishizawa T, Kato T, Matsuura T, Sato S, Tamura T, Higuchi Y, Watanabe T, Kitamura H, Asanuma K, Yamazaki T, Ikemi M, Kitagawa H, Morikawa T, Ikeya H, Maeda K, Takahashi K, Nohmi K, Izutani N, Kanda M, Suzuki R. Novel hyaluronic acid-methotrexate conjugates for osteoarthritis treatment. *Biorganic Medicinal Chemistry* 2009;17:4647-56.

Hooper L, Brown TJ, Elliott R, Payne K, Roberts C, Symmons D. The effectiveness of five strategies for the prevention of gastrointestinal toxicity induced by non-steroidal anti-inflammatory drugs: systematic review. *BMJ* 2004;329:948-58.

Huerta C, Castellsague J, Varas-Lorenzo C, García Rodríguez LA. Nonsteroidal anti-inflammatory drugs and risk of ARF in the general population *Am. J. Kidney Dis.* 2005;45:531-9.

Hunter DJ, Le Graverand MP, Eckstein F. Radiologic markers of osteoarthritis progression. *Curr. Opin. Rheumatol.* 2009;21:110-7.

Hunter DJ, Pharmacologic therapy for osteoarthritis--the era of disease modification.*Nat. Rev. Rheumatol.* 2011;7:13-22.

Huskisson EC, Berry H, Gishen P, Jubb RW, Whitehead J. Effects of antiinflammatory drugs on the progression of osteoarthritis of the knee. LINK Study Group. Longitudinal investigation of nonsteroidal antiinflamatory drugs in knee osteoarthritis. *J. Rheumatol*, 1995;22:1941–6.

Israel HA, Ramamiurthy NS, Greenwald R, Golub L. The Potential Role of Doxycycline in the Treatment of Osteoarthritis of the Temporomandibular Joint. *Adv. Dent Res.* 1998;12:51-5.

Jordan KM, Arden NK, Doherty M, Bannwarth B, Bijlsma JW, Dieppe P, Gunther K, Hauselmann H, Herrero-Beaumont G, Kaklamanis P, Lohmander S, Leeb B, Lequesne M, Mazieres B, Martin-Mola E, Pavelka K, Pendleton A, Punzi L, Serni U, Swoboda B, Verbruggen G, Zimmerman-Gorska I, Dougados M; Standing Committee for International Clinical Studies EULAR Recommendations 2003: an evidence based approach to the management of knee osteoarthritis: Report of a Task Force of the Standing Committee for International Clinical Studies Including Therapeutic Trials (ESCISIT). *Ann. Rheum. Dis.* 2003;62:1145-55.

Jovanovic DV, Fernandes JC, Martel-Pelletier J, Jolicoeur FC, Reboul P, Laufer S, Tries S, Pelletier JP. The in vivo dual inhibition of cyclooxygenase and lipoxygenase by ML-3000 reduces the progression of experimental osteoarthritis. Suppression of collagenase-1 and interleukin-1beta synthesis. *Arthritis Rheum.* 2001;44:2320–30.

Jüni P, Nartey L, Reichenbach S, Sterchi R, Dieppe PA, Egger M. Risk of cardiovascular events and rofecoxib: cumulative meta-analysis. *Lancet* 2004; 364: 2021-9.

Jüni P, Reichenbach S, Trelle S, Tschannen B, Wandel S, Jordi B, Züllig M, Guetg R, Häuselmann HJ, Schwarz H, Theiler R, Ziswiler HR, Dieppe PA, Villiger PM, Egger M; Swiss Viscosupplementation Trial Group. Efficacy and safety of intraarticular hylan or hyaluronic acids for osteoarthritis of the knee: a randomized controlled trial. *Arthritis Rheum* 2007;56:3610-9.

Kadam UT, Jordan K, Croft PR. Clinical comorbidity in patients with osteoarthritis: a casecontrol study of general practice consulters in England and Wales. *Ann. Rheum. Dis.* 2004;63:408–14.

Karlsson J, Pivodic A, Aguirre D, Schnitzer TJ. Efficacy, safety and tolerability of the cyclooxygenase-inhibiting nitric oxide donator naproxcinod in treating osteoarthritis of the hip or knee. *J. Rheumatol* 2009;36:1290-7.

Kearney PM, Baigent C, Godwin J, Halls H, Emberson JR, Patrono C, Do selective cyclo-oxygenase-2 inhibitors and traditional non-steroidal anti-inflammatory drugs increase the risk of atherothrombosis? Meta-analysis of randomised trials. *BMJ* 2006;332:1302-8.

Klesser B, Bias P, Buchner A, Elsaesser R. Licofelone (ML3000), an inhibitor of COX-1, COX-2 and 5-LOX, has little or no effect on the gastric mucosa after 4 weeks of treatment. *Ann. Rheum Dis*, 2002;61(Suppl. 1):130.

Krzeski P, Buckland-Wright C, Bálint G, Cline GA, Stoner K, Lyon R, Beary J, Aronstein WS, Spector TD. Development of musculoskeletal toxicity without clear benefit after administration of PG-116800, a matrix metalloproteinase inhibitor, to patients with knee osteoarthritis: a randomized, 12-month, double-blind, placebo-controlled study. *Arthritis Res. Ther* 2007; 9(5): R109.

Lanas A, Tornero J, Zamorano JL. Assessment of gastrointestinal and cardiovascular risk in patients with osteoarthritis who require NSAIDs: the LOGICA study. *Ann. Rheum. Dis.* 2010;69:1453-8.

Langford R, McKenna F, Ratcliffe S, Vojtassák J. Transdermal fentanyl for improvement of pain and functioning in osteoarthritis: a randomized, placebo-controlled trial. *Arthritis Rheum* 2006;54:1829-37.

Latimer N, Lord J, Grant RL, O'Mahony R, Dickson J, Conaghan PG; National Institute for Health and Clinical Excellence Osteoarthritis Guideline Development Group. Cost effectiveness of COX 2 selective inhibitors and traditional NSAIDs alone or in combination with a proton pump inhibitor for people with osteoarthritis. *BMJ* 2009;339:b2538.

Lawrence RC, Felson DT, Helmick CG, Arnold LM, Choi H, Deyo RA, Gabriel S, Hirsch R, Hochberg MC, Hunder GG, Jordan JM, Katz JN, Kremers HM, Wolfe F; National Arthritis Data Workgroup. Estimates of the prevalence of arthritis and other rheumatic conditions in the United States. *Part II. Arthritis Rheum* 2008;58:26-35.

Leeb BF, Schweitzer H, Montag K, Smolen JS. A metaanalysis of chondroitin sulfate in the treatment of osteoarthritis. *J. Rheumatol.* 2000;27:205-11

Lethbridge-Cejku M, Helmick CG, Popovic JR. Hospitalizations for arthritis and other rheumatic conditions: data from the 1997 National Hospital Discharge Survey. *Med Care.* 2003;41: 1367-73.

Levy D, Zochodne DW. Increased mRNA expression of the B1 and B2 bradykinin receptors and antinociceptive effects of their antagonists in an animal model of neuropathic pain. *Pain* 2000;86:265–71.

Lewis EJ, Bishop J, Bottomley KM, Bradshaw D, Brewster M, Broadhurst MJ, Brown PA, Budd JM, Elliott L, Greenham AK, Johnson WH, Nixon JS, Rose F, Sutton B, Wilson K. Ro 32-3555, an orally active collagenase inhibitor, prevents cartilage breakdown in vitro and in vivo. *Br. J. Pharmacol.* 1997; 121:540-6.

Lo GH, LaValley M, McAlindon T, Felson DT. Intra-articular hyaluronic acid in treatment of knee osteoarthritis: a meta-analysis. *JAMA* 2003;290:3115-21.

Lohmander LS, McKeith D, Svensson O, Malmenas M, Bolin L, Kalla A, Genti G, Szechinski J, Ramos-Remus C; STAR Multinational Study Group. A randomised, placebo controlled, comparative trial of the gastrointestinal safety and efficacy of AZD3582 versus naproxen in osteoarthritis. *Ann. Rheum. Dis.* 2005;64:449–56.

Magnano MD ,Chakravarty EF, Broudy C, Chung L, Kelman A, Hillygus J, Genovese MC. A pilot study of tumor necrosis factor inhibition in erosive/inflammatory osteoarthritis of the hands. *J. Rheumatol.* 2007 Jun; 34: 1323-7.

Mannoni A, Altman R, Muniz OE, Serni U, Dean DD. The effects of methotrexate on normal and osteoarthritic lapine articular cartilage. *J. Rheumatol.* 1993;20:849-855.

Marceau F, Regoli D. Bradykinin receptor ligands: therapeutic perspectives. *Nat Rev Drug Discov* 2004;3:845–52.

Marcouiller P, Pelletier JP, Guıvremont M, Martel-Pelletier J, Ranger P, Laufer S, Reboul P. Leukotriene and prostaglandin synthesis pathways in osteoarthritic synovial membranes: regulating factors for IL-1beta synthesis. *J. Rheumatol.,* 2005;32:704–12.

Marks R, Allegrante JP. Comorbid disease profiles of adults with end-stage hip osteoarthritis. *Med. Sci. Monit.* 2002;8:CR305-9.

Martel-Pelletier J, Lajeunesse D, Reboul P, Pelletier JP. Therapeutic role of dual inhibitors of 5-LOX and COX, selective and nonselective nonsteroidal anti-inflammatory drugs. *Ann. Rheum. Dis.,* 2003;62:501–9.

Martel-Pelletier J, Mineau F, Jolicoeur FC, Cloutier JM, Pelletier JP. In vitro effects of diacerhein and rhein on interleukin 1 and tumor necrosis factor-alpha systems in human osteoarthritic synovium and chondrocytes. *J. Rheumatol.* 1998;25:753-62.

Mazzuca SA, Brandt KD, Katz BP, Lane KA, Bradley JD, Heck LW, Hugenberg ST, Manzi S, Moreland LW, Oddis CV, Schnitzer TJ, Sharma L, Wolfe F, Yocum DE. Subject retention and adherence in a randomized placebo-controlled trial of a disease-modifying osteoarthritis drug. *Arthritis Rheum*; 51: 933–940.

Mc Alindon TE, LaValley MP, Gulin JP, Felson DT. Glucosamine and chondroitin for treatment of osteoarthritis: a systematic quality assessment and meta-analysis. *JAMA* 2000;283:1469-75.

Moldovan F, Pelletier JP, Jolicoeur FC, Cloutier JM, Martel-Pelletier J. Diacerhein and rhein reduce the ICE-induced IL-1beta and IL-18 activation in human osteoarthritic cartilage. *Osteoarthritis Cartilage* 2000;8:186-96.

Momi S, Emerson M, Paul W, Leone M, Mezzasoma AM, Del Soldato P, Page CP, Gresele P. Prevention of pulmonary thromboembolism by NCX 4016, a nitric oxide-releasing aspirin. *Eur. J. Pharmacol.* 2000;397: 177–85

Moore RA, Tramèr MR, Carroll D, Wiffen PJ, McQuay HJ. Quantitative systematic review of topically applied non-steroidal anti-inflammatory drugs. *BMJ* 1998;316:333-8.

Muscará MN, Lovren F, McKnight W, Dicay M, del Soldato P, Triggle CR, Wallace JL. Vasorelaxant effects of a nitric oxide releasing aspirin derivative in normotensive and hypertensive rats. *Br. J. Pharmacol.* 2001;133: 1314–22.

Muscará MN, McKnight W, Del Soldato P, Wallace JL. Effect of a nitric oxide-releasing naproxen derivative on hypertension and gastric damage induced by chronic nitric oxide inhibition in the rat. *Life Sci.* 1998;62: PL235–PL240

Muscará MN, McKnight W, Lovren F, Triggle CR, Cirino G, Wallace JL. Antihypertensive properties of a nitric oxide-releasing naproxen derivative in two-kidney, one-clip rats. *Am. J. Physiol. Heart Circ. Physiol.* 2000;279: H528–H535.

Neidel J, Schroers B, Sintermann F. The effects of high-dose methotrexate on the development of cartilage lesions in a lapine model of osteoarthritis. *Arch. Orthop Trauma Surg.* 1998;117:265-9.

Nickles CJ, Yelland M, Del Mar C, Wilkinson D, The role of paracetamol in chronic pain: an evidence-based approach. *Am. J. Ther.* 2005;12:80-91.

Nishimura M, Segami N, Kaneyama K, Suzuki T, Miyamaru M. Relationships between pain-related mediators and both synovitis and joint pain in patients with internal derangements and osteoarthritis of the temporomandibular joint. *Oral Surg Oral Med Oral Pathol Oral Radiol Endod.* 2002;94:328–32.

Nüesch E, Reichenbach S, Trelle S, Rutjes AW, Liewald K, Sterchi R, Altman DG, Jüni P.The importance of allocation concealment and patient blinding in osteoarthritis trials: a meta-epidemiologic study. *Arthritis Rheum* 2009a;61:1633-41.

Nüesch E, Rutjes AWS, Husni E,Welch V, Jüni P. Oral or transdermal opioids for osteoarthritis of the knee or hip. *Cochrane Database Syst Rev* 2009b;(4): CD003115.

Nüesch E, Rutjes AWS, Trelle S, Reichenbach S, Jüni P. Doxycycline for osteoarthritis of the knee or hip. *Cochrane Database of Systematic Reviews* 2009c; 4: CD007323.

Nüesch E, Trelle S, Reichenbach S, Rutjes AW, Tschannen B, Altman DG, Egger M, Jüni P. Small study effects in meta-analyses of osteoarthritis trials: meta-epidemiological study. *BMJ* 2010;341:c3515.

Onel E, Kolsun K, Kauffman JI. Post-Hoc analysis of a head-to-head hyaluronic acid comparison in knee osteoarthritis using the 2004 OMERACT-OARSI responder criteria. *Clin. Drug Investig.* 2008;28:37-45.

Pal B, Morris J. Perceived risks of joint infection following intra-articular corticosteroid injections: a survey of rheumatologists. *Clin. Rheumatol.* 1999;18:264-5.

Parades Y, Massicotte F, Pelletier JP, Martel-Pelletier J, Laufer S, Lajeunesse D. Study of the role of leukotriene B( )4 in abnormal function of human subchondral osteoarthritis osteoblasts: effects of cyclooxygenase and/or 5-lipoxygenase inhibition. *Arthritis Rheum*, 2002;46:1804–1812.

Parmigiani L, Furtado RN, Lopes RV, Ribeiro LH, Natour J. Joint lavage associated with triamcinolone hexacetonide injection in knee osteoarthritis: a randomized double-blind controlled study. *Clin. Rheumatol.* 2010;29:1311-5.

Patrono C, Non-steroidal anti-inflammatory drugs. Rheumatology, 4th ed,2007, Mosby, Eds Hochberg MC, Silman AJ, Smolen JS, Weinblatt ME, Weisman MH. pp 403-10.

Pavelka K, Bias P, Buchner A, et al. Licofelone, an inhibitor of COX-1, COX-2 and 5-LOX, is as effective as celecoxib and shows improved tolerability during 12 weeks of treatment in patients with osteoarthritis of the knee. *Ann. Rheum Dis*, 2003; 62(Suppl. 1):261.

Pelletier JP, Boileau C, Brunet J, Boily M, Lajeunesse D, Reboul P, Laufer S, Martel-Pelletier J. The inhibition of subchondral bone resorption in the early phase of experimental dog osteoarthritis by licofelone is associated with a reduction in the synthesis of MMP-13 and cathepsin K. *Bone* 2004;34:527–538.

Pelletier JP, Caron JP, Evans C, Robbins PD, Georgescu HI, Jovanovic D, Fernandes JC, Martel-Pelletier J.. In vivo suppression of early experimental osteoarthritis by interleukin-1 receptor antagonist using gene therapy. *Arthritis Rheum.* 1997;40:1012-9.

Pergolizzi J, Böger RH, Budd K, Dahan A, Erdine S, Hans G, Kress HG, Langford R, Likar R, Raffa RB, Sacerdote P, Opioids and the management of chronic severe pain in the elderly: consensus statement of an International Expert Panel with focus on the six clinically most often used World Health Organization Step III opioids (buprenorphine, fentanyl, hydromorphone, methadone, morphine, oxycodone). *Pain Pract* 2008;8:287-313.

Perkins MN, Campbell E, Dray A. Antinociceptive activity of the bradykinin B1 and B2 receptor antagonists, des-Arg9, [Leu8]-BK and HOE 140, in two models of persistent hyperalgesia in the rat. *Pain* 1993;53:191–7.

Pham T, Le Henanff A, Ravaud P, Dieppe P, Paolozzi L, Dougados M. Evaluation of the symptomatic and structural efficacy of a new hyaluronic acid compound, NRD101, in comparison with diacerein and placebo in a 1 year randomised controlled study in symptomatic knee osteoarthritis. *Ann Rheum. Dis.* 2004;63:1611-17.

Pincus T, Koch GG, Sokka T, Lefkowith J, Wolfe F, Jordan JM, Luta G, Callahan LF, Wang X, Schwartz T, Abramson SB, Caldwell JR, Harrell RA, Kremer JM, Lautzenheiser RL, Markenson JA, Schnitzer TJ, Weaver A, Cummins P, Wilson A, Morant S, Fort J. A randomized, double-blind, crossover clinical trial of diclofenac plus misoprostol versus acetaminophen in patients with osteoarthritis of the hip or knee. *Arthritis Rheum.* 2001;44:1587-98.

Presotto C, Bolla MI, Olivieri R, Schnitzer TJ, Wallace JL. HCT 3012 reduces blood pressure in the spontaneously hypertensive rat model. *Arthritis Rheum.* 2006;54(suppl 9): S147.

Punzi L, Bertazzolo N, Pianon M, Michelotto M, Todesco S. Soluble interleukin 2 receptors and treatment with hydroxychloroquine in erosive osteoarthritis. *J. Rheumatol.* 1996;23:1477-8.

Rainsford KD, Ying C, Smith F. Effects of 5-lipoxygenase inhibitors on interleukin production by human synovial tissues in organ culture: comparison with interleukin-1-synthesis inhibitors. *J. Pharm. Pharmacol,* 1996;48:46–52.

Ravauld P, Moulinier L, Giraudeau B, Ayral X, Guerin C, Noel E, Thomas P, Fautrel B, Mazieres B, Dougados M. Effects of joint lavage and steroid injection in patients with osteoarthritis of the knee: results of a multicenter, randomized, controlled trial. *Arthritis Rheum* 1999;42:475-82.

Raynauld JP, Buckland-Wright C, Ward R, Choquette D, Haraoui B, Martel-Pelletier J, Uthman I, Khy V, Tremblay JL, Bertrand C, Pelletier JP. Safety and efficacy of long-term intraarticular steroid injections in osteoarthritis of the knee: a randomized, double-blind, placebo-controlled trial. *Arthritis Rheum.* 2003;48:370-7.

Raynauld JP, Martel-Pelletier J, Raynauld JP, Martel-Pelletier J, Bias P, Laufer S, Haraoui B, Choquette D, Beaulieu AD, Abram F, Dorais M, Vignon E, Pelletier JP; Canadian Licofelone Study Group. Protective effects of licofelone, a 5-lipoxygenase and cyclo-oxygenase inhibitor, verus naproxen, in cartilage loss in knee osteoarthritis: a first multicentre clinical trial using quantitative MRI. *Ann. Rheum Dis.* 2009; 68: 938-47.

Reginster JY, Bias P, Buchner A. First clinical results of licofelone (ML3000), an inhibitor of COX-1, COX-2 and 5-LOX, for the treatment of osteoarthritis. *Ann. Rheum Dis,* 2002; 61(Suppl. 1):116–7.

Regoli D, Nsa Allogho S, Rizzi A, Gobeil FJ. Bradykinin receptors and their antagonists. *Eur. J. Pharmacol.* 1998;348:1–10.

Reichenbach S, Blank S, Rutjes AW, Shang A, King EA, Dieppe PA, Jüni P, Trelle S. Hylan versus hyaluronic acid for osteoarthritis of the knee: a systematic review and meta-analysis. *Arthritis Rheum* 2007a;57:1410-8.

Reichenbach S, Sterchi R, Scherer M, Trelle S, Bürgi E, Bürgi U, Dieppe PA, Jüni P. Meta-analysis: chondroitin for osteoarthritis of the knee or hip. *Ann. Intern. Med.* 2007b;146:580-90.

Rhaleb NE, Rouissi N, Jukic D, Regoli D, Henke S, Breipohl G, Knolle J. Pharmacological characterization of a new highly potent B2 receptor antagonist (HOE 140: D-Arg- [Hyp3,Thi5,D-Tic7,Qic8]bradykinin). *Eur. J. Pharmacol.* 1992;210:115–20.

Richy F, Bruyere O, Ethgen O, Cucherat M, Henrotin Y, Reginster JY. Structural and symptomatic efficacy of glucosamine and chondroitin in knee osteoarthritis: a comprehensive meta-analysis. *Arch. Intern. Med.* 2003;163:1514-22.

Rintelen B, Neumann K, Leeb BF. A meta-analysis of controlled clinical studies with diacerein in the treatment of osteoarthritis. *Arch. Intern. Med.* 2006;166:1899-906.

Roberts WN, Babcock EA, Breitbach SA, Owen DS, Irby WR. Corticosteroid injection in rheumatoid arthritis does not increase rate of total joint arthroplasty. *J. Rheumatol.* 1996;23:1001-4.

Rossoni G, Manfredi B, De Gennaro Colonna V, Brini AT, Polvani G, Clement MG, Berti F. Nitric oxide and prostacyclin pathways: an integrated mechanism that limits myocardial infraction progression in anaesthetized rats. *Pharmacol. Res* 2006; 53: 359-366.

Rossoni G. Manfredi B, Del Soldato P, Berti F. The nitric oxide-releasing naproxen derivative displays cardioprotection in perfused rabbit heart submitted to ischemia-reperfusion. *J. Pharmacol. Exp. Ther.* 2004;310: 555–562

Sacks JJ, Helmick CG, Langmaid G, Deaths from arthritis and other rheumatic conditions, United States, 1979-1998. *J. Rheumatol.* 2004;31:1823–1828.

Sadreddini S, Noshad H, Molaeefard M, Moloudi R, Ardalan MR, Ghojazadeh M. A double blind, randomized, placebo controlled study to evaluate the efficacy of erythromycin in patients with knee effusion due to osteoarthritis. *Int. J. Rheum. Dis.* 2009; 12(1): 44-51.

Schafer PH, Parton A, Gandhi AK, Capone L, Adams M, Wu L, Bartlett JB, Loveland MA, Gilhar A, Cheung Y-F, Baillie GS, Houslay MD, Man H-W, Muller GW, Stirling D. Apremilast, a cAMP phosphodiesterase-4 inhibitor, demonstrates anti-inflammatory activity in vitro and in a model of psoriasis. *British Journal of Pharmacology* 2010; 159:842-855.

Schnitzer TJ, Burmester GR, Mysler E, Hochberg MC, Doherty M, Ehrsam E, Gitton X, Krammer G, Mellein B, Matchaba P, Gimona A, Hawkey CJ; TARGET Study Group. Comparison of lumiracoxib with naproxen and ibuprofen in the Therapeutic Arthritis Research and Gastrointestinal Event Trial (TARGET), reduction in ulcer complications: randomised controlled trial. *Lancet* 2004;364:665-74.

Schnitzer TJ, Hochber MC, Marrero CE, Duquesroix B, Frayssinet H, Beekman M. Efficacy and safety of naproxcinod in patients with osteoarthritis of the knee: a 53-week prospective randomized multicenter study. *Semin Arthritis Rheum* 2011;40:285-297.

Schnitzer TJ, Kamin M, Olson WH. Tramadol allows reduction of naproxen dose among patients with naproxen-responsive osteoarthritis pain: a randomized, double-blind, placebo-controlled study. *Arthritis Rheum* 1999;42:1370-7.

Schnitzer TJ, Kivitz A, Frayssinet H, Duquesroix B. Efficacy and safety of naproxcinod in the treatment of patients with osteoarthritis of the knee: a 13-week prospective, randomized, multicenter study. *Osteoarthritis Cartilage* 2010;18:629-639.

Schnitzer TJ, Kivitz AJ, Lipetz RS, Sanders N, Hee A. Comparison of the COX-inhibiting nitric oxide donor AZD3582 and rofecoxib in treating the signs and symptoms of osteoarthritis of the knee. *Arthritis Rheum.* 2005;53: 827–837

Schoenfeld A, Bar Y, Merlob P, Ovadia Y. NSAIDs: maternal and fetal considerations. *Am. J. Reprod. Immunol.* 1992;3-4:141-7.

Schumacher HR, Chen LX. Injectable corticosteroids in treatment of arthritis of the knee. *Am. J. Med.* 2005;118:1208-14.

Sekut L, Yarnall D, Stimpson SA, Noel LS, Bateman-Fite R, Clark RL, Brackeen MF, Menius JA Jr, Connolly KM. Anti-inflammatory activity of phosphodiesterase (PDE)-IV inhibitors in acute and chronic models of inflammation. *Clin. Exp. Immunol.* 1995; 100:126-132.

Sharma JN, Wirth KJ. Inhibition of rats adjuvant arthritis by a bradykinin antagonist Hoe 140 and its influence on kallikreins. *Gen. Pharmacol.* 1996;27:133–136.

Singh G, Miller ID, Lee FH, Pettitt D, Russell MW. Prevalence of cardiovascular disease risk factors among US adults with self-reported osteoarthritis: data from the Third National Health and Nutrition Examination Survey. *Am. J. Manag Care.* 2002;8(15 suppl): S383-S391.

Singh JA, Mahowald ML, Noorbaloochi S. Intra-articular botulinum toxin A for refractory shoulder pain: a randomized, double-blinded, placebo-controlled trial. *Transl Res* 2009;153:205–216.

Singh JA. Botulinum toxin therapy for osteoartricular pain: an evidence-based review. *Ther. Adv. Musculoskelet Dis.* 2010; 2(2): 105-118.

Singh VP, Patil CS, Kulkarni SK. Anti-inflammatory effect of licofelone against various inflammatory challenges. *Fundam Clin. Pharmacol*, 2006;20:65–71.

Song IH, Althoff CE, Hermann KG, Scheel AK, Knetsch T, Burmester GR, Backhaus M. Contrast-enhanced ultrasound in monitoring the efficacy of a bradykinin receptor 2 antagonist in painful knee osteoarthritis compared with MRI. *Ann. Rheum. Dis.* 2009; 68:75-83.

Stürmer T, Sun Y, Sauerland S, Zeissig I, Günther KP, Puhl W, etal. Serum cholesterol and osteoarthritis. The baseline examination of the Ulm Osteoarthritis Study. *J. Rheumatol.* 1998;25:1827-32.

Swan SK, Rudy DW, Lasseter KC, Ryan CF, Buechel KL, Lambrecht LJ, Pinto MB, Dilzer SC, Obrda O, Sundblad KJ, Gumbs CP, Ebel DL, Quan H, Larson PJ, Schwartz JI, Musliner TA, Gertz BJ, Brater DC, Yao SL. Effect of cyclooxygenase-2 inhibition on renal function in elderly persons receiving a low-salt diet. A randomized, controlled trial. *Ann. Intern. Med.* 2000;133:1-9.

Temple AR, Benson GD, Zinsenheim JR, Schweinle JE. Multicenter, randomized, double-blind, active-controlled, parallel-group trial of the long-term (6-12 months) safety of acetaminophen in adult patients with osteoarthritis. *Clin. Ther.* 2006;28:222-35.

Tonussi CR, Ferreira SH. Bradykinin-induced knee joint incapacitation involves bradykinin B2 receptor mediated hyperalgesia and bradykinin B1 receptor-mediated nociception. *Eur. J. Pharmacol.* 1997;326:61–65.

Towheed T, Maxwell L, Anastassiades TP, Shea B, Houpt JB, Welch V, Hochberg MC, Wells GA. Glucosamine therapy for treating osteoarthritis. *Cochrane Database of Syst Rev.* 2005;(2): CD002946.

Towheed TE, Maxwell L, Judd MG, Catton M, Hochberg MC, Wells G. Acetaminophen for osteoarthritis. *Cochrane Database Syst Rev.* 2009 (1):CD004257.

Towheed TE, Pennsaid therapy for osteoarthritis of the knee: a systematic review and metaanalysis of randomized controlled trials. *J. Rheumatol* 2006;33:567-73.

Trelle S, Reichenbach S, Wandel S, Hildebrand P, Tschannen B, Villiger PM, Egger M, Cardiovascular safety of non-steroidal anti-inflammatory drugs: network meta-analysis. *BMJ* 2011;342:c7086.

Tugwell PS, Wells GA, Shainhouse JZ Equivalence study of a topical diclofenac solution (pennsaid) compared with oral diclofenac in symptomatic treatment of osteoarthritis of the knee: a randomized controlled trial. *J. Rheumatol* 2004;31:2002-12.

Vestergaard P, Rejnmark L, Mosekilde L, Fracture risk associated with the use of morphine and opiates. *J. Intern. Med* 2006;260:76-87.

Vuolteenaho K, Kujala P, Moilanen T, Moilanen E. Aurothiomalate and hydroxychloroquine inhibit nitric oxide production in chondrocytes and in human osteoarthritic cartilage. *Scand. J. Rheumatol.* 2005; 34: 475-9.

Wada J, Koshino T, Morii T, Sugimoto K. Natural course of osteoarthritis of the knee treated with or without intraarticular corticosteroid injections. *Bull Hosp Joint Dis* 1993;53:45-8.

Wallace JL, Carter L, McKnight W, Tries S, Laufer S. ML 3000 reduces gastric prostaglandin synthesis without causing mucosal injury. *Eur. J. Pharmacol,* 1994b;271:525–31.

Wallace JL, McKnight W, Del Soldato P, Baydoun AR, Cirino G.. Anti-thrombotic effects of a nitric oxide releasing, gastric-sparing aspirin derivative. *J. Clin. Invest.* 1995;96: 2711– 8.

Wallace JL, Reuter B, Cicala C, McKnight W, Grisham M, Cirino G. A diclofenac derivative without ulcerogenic properties. *Eur. J. Pharmacol.* 1994a; 257:249–55.

Wallace JL, Reuter B, Cicala C, McKnight W, Grisham MB, Cirino G. Novel nonsteroidal anti-inflammatory drug derivatives with markedly reduced ulcerogenic properties in the rat. *Gastroenterology* 1994c; 107: 173–9.

Wallace JL, Viappiani S, Bolla M. Cyclooxygenase-inhibiting nitric oxide donators for osteoarthritis. *Trends Pharmacol Sci* 2009; 30: 112-7.

Wandel S, Jüni P, Tendal B, Nüesch E, Villiger PM, Welton NJ, Reichenbach S, Trelle S. Effects of glucosamine, chondroitin, or placebo in patients with osteoarthritis of hip or knee: network meta-analysis. *BMJ* 2010;341:c4675.

Wanders A, Heijde D, Landewé R, Béhier JM, Calin A, Olivieri I, Zeidler H, Dougados M. Nonsteroidal antiinflammatory drugs reduce radiographic progression in patients with ankylosing spondylitis: a randomized clinical trial. *Arthritis Rheum* 2005;52:1756-65.

Wang CT, Lin J, Chang CJ, Lin YT, Hou SM. Therapeutic effects of hyaluronic acid on osteoarthritis of the knee. A meta-analysis of randomized controlled trials. *J. Bone Joint Surg* 2004;86-A:538-45.

West PM, Fernandez C. Safety of COX-2 inhibitors in asthma patients with aspirin hypersensitivity. *Ann. Pharmacother* 2003;37:1497-1501.

White WB, Schnitzer TJ, Bakris GL, Frayssinet H, Duquesroix B, Weber M. Effects of Naproxcinod on blood pressure in patients with osteoarthritis. *Am. J. Cardiol*. 2011; [ahead of print].

White WB, Schnitzer TJ, Fleming R, Duquesroix B, Beekman M. Effects of the cyclooxygenase inhibiting nitric oxide donator naproxcinod versus naproxen on systemic blood pressure in patients with osteoarthritis. *Am. J. Card*. 2009;840–5.

WHO Expert Commitee on Drug Dependence, Thirty-fourth report, 2008, available at http://whqlibdoc.who.int/trs/WHO_TRS_942_eng.pdf.

Wilson PWF, D' Agostino RB, Levy D, Belanger AM, Silbershatz H, Kannel WB. Prediction of coronary heart disease using risk factor categories. *Circulation* 1998;97:1837-47.

Wu CW, Terkeltaub R, Kalunian KC, Calcium-containing crystals and osteoarthritis: implications for the clinician. *Curr. Rheumatol. Rep.* 2005;7:213-9.

Zhang W, Doherty M, Arden N, Bannwarth B, Bijlsma J, Gunther KP, Hauselmann HJ, Herrero-Beaumont G, Jordan K, Kaklamanis P, Leeb B, Lequesne M, Lohmander S, Mazieres B, Martin-Mola E, Pavelka K, Pendleton A, Punzi L, Swoboda B, Varatojo R, Verbruggen G, Zimmermann-Gorska I, Dougados M; EULAR Standing Committee for International Clinical Studies Including Therapeutics (ESCISIT). EULAR evidence based recommendations for the management of hip osteoarthritis: report of a task force of the EULAR Standing Committee for International Clinical Studies Including Therapeutics (ESCISIT). *Ann Rheum. Dis*. 2005;64:669-81.

Zhang W, Doherty M, Leeb BF, Alekseeva L, Arden NK, Bijlsma JW, Dinçer F, Dziedzic K, Häuselmann HJ, Herrero-Beaumont G, Kaklamanis P, Lohmander S, Maheu E, Martín-Mola E, Pavelka K, Punzi L, Reiter S, Sautner J, Smolen J, Verbruggen G, Zimmermann-Górska I. EULAR evidence based recommendations for the management of hand osteoarthritis: report of a Task Force of the EULAR Standing Committee for International Clinical Studies Including Therapeutics (ESCISIT). *Ann Rheum. Dis*. 2007;66:377-88.

Zhang W, Jones A, Doherty M. Does paracetamol (acetaminophen) reduce the pain of osteoarthritis? A meta-analysis of randomised controlled trials. *Ann. Rheum. Dis.* 2004;63:901-7.

Zhang W, Moskowitz RW, Nuki G, Abramson S, Altman RD, Arden N, Bierma-Zeinstra S, Brandt KD, Croft P, Doherty M, Dougados M, Hochberg M, Hunter DJ, Kwoh K, Lohmander LS, Tugwell P. OARSI recommendations for the management of hip and knee osteoarthritis, Part II: OARSI evidence-based, expert consensus guidelines. *Osteoarthritis Cartilage* 2008a;16:137-62.

Zhang W, Robertson J, Jones AC, Dieppe PA, Doherty M. The placebo effect and its determinants in osteoarthritis: meta-analysis of randomised controlled trials. *Ann. Rheum. Dis.* 2008b;67:1716-23.

Zhang X, Schwarz EM, Young DA, Puzas JE, Rosier RN, O'Keefe RJ. Cyclooxygenase-2 regulates mesenchymal cell differentiation into the osteoblast lineage and is critically involved in bone repair. *J. Clin. Invest* 2002;109:1405-15.

In: Arthritis: Types, Treatment and Prevention   ISBN 978-1-61470-719-6
Editor: Marc N. Pelt   © 2012 Nova Science Publishers, Inc.

Chapter II

Psoriatic Arthritis: Types, Health Effects and Treatments

*J. A. O'Daly**

Astralis Ltd,. Irvington,
New Jersey. US

ABSTRACT

Psoriatic arthritis (PsA) types are described following the
CLASsification of Psoriatic ARthritis (CASPAR) criteria, after the
classic paper published by Moll and Wright in 1973. The PsA types can
be summarized as: 1- Evidence of psoriasis (a) Current psoriatic skin or
scalp disease (b) Personal history of psoriasis (c) Family history of
psoriasis 2- Psoriatic nail dystrophy including onycholysis, pitting and
hyperkeratosis 3 - A negative test for rheumatoid factor. 4 - Dactylitis 5 -
Radiological evidence of juxta-articular new bone formation. A
description of prevalence and incidence is presented, analyzing disease
importance in the world. The relationship between psoriasis and PsA is
analyzed from the genetic point of view. In psoriasis, the association is
with class I antigens: HLAB13, HLA-B17, HLACw6, and HLA-Cw7.
The allele HLA-Cw602 is associated with early onset of psoriasis, higher
incidence of guttate or streptococcal induced disease flares, and more

* Corresponding author: J.A. O'Daly. Tel: 973-224-5723. email: joseodaly@aol.com

severe disease. The allele HLA-B27 is associated with greater spinal involvement, while B38 and B39 are associated with peripheral polyarthritis. In contrast to rheumatoid arthritis (RA), the joint distribution in PsA tends to be asymmetrical and oligoarticular (< five joints). Distal joints, particularly the distal interphalangeal (DIP) joints of the hands, are more frequently affected; joint tenderness tends to be less; and dactylitis, enthesitis and axial or spinal involvement are more frequent. PsA includes the absence of rheumatoid nodules, of rheumatoid factor in the blood and in some instances presence of iritis, mucous membrane lesions, urethritis, bowel inflammation and tendonitis. Patients with PsA have an increased incidence of cardiovascular disease (CVD) and cardiovascular risk factors such as smoking, hypertension, and metabolic syndrome compared to the normal population. In patients with PsA, carotid wave pulse velocity, a measure of arterial stiffness, is significantly higher as is subclinical atherosclerosis as measured by arterial intima-media wall thickness (IMT) and endothelial dysfunction. Therapies that target cells, such as activated T cells, and proinflammatory cytokines, such as tumor necrosis factor alpha (TNFα), are current treatments in use today. Traditional therapies for PsA like nonsteroidal anti-inflammatory drugs (NSAIDs), oral immunomodulatory drugs, topical creams, and light therapy have been helpful in controlling both musculoskeletal and dermatologic lesions of the disease, but may eventually show diminished benefit, and may produce severe toxicities as side effects. A first generation polyvalent vaccine, with leishmania amastigotes antigens, from 4 leishmania species has been found to decrease psoriasis and PsA, in several human clinical trials. Also mice collagen induced arthritis decreased markedly after treatment with purified leishmania antigens. Their antigenic effect has been explained by immunomodulation of T and B cells not by immunosuppression contrary to existing treatments on the market today.

INTRODUCTION

Psoriatic Arthritis Types

The first description of PsA is attributed to Louis Aliberti, who in 1818 first noted the relationship between psoriasis and arthritis. Pierre Bazin then described "Psoriasis Arthritique" in 1860, followed by Charles Bourdillon in 1888 with "Psoriasis et Arthropathies". Jeghers and Robinson in 1937, and Vilanova and Piñol in 1951 described PsA as a unique entity [1].

All studies of PsA use the criteria by Moll and Wright in their classic paper published in 1973: A- presence of psoriasis, B- inflammatory arthritis and C- negative test for rheumatoid factor. The PsA subgroups described with these criteria were: 1- Distal interphalangeal (DIP) joint disease (5%); 2- Asymmetrical oligoarthritis (70%); 3- Polyarthritis (15%); 4- Spondylitis (5%); 5- Arthritis mutilans (5%) [2]. Gladman expanded the five sub-groups to seven: Distal disease (DIP only affected), oligoarthritis (<4 joints), polyarthritis, spondylitis only, distal disease plus spondylitis, oligoarthritis plus spondylitis and polyarthritis plus spondylitis [3].

The prevalence and incidence estimates of psoriasis and PsA show ethnic and geographic variations, being generally more common in the colder north than in the tropics. In Europe the prevalence of psoriasis varies anywhere from 0.6 to 6.5%. In the USA, the prevalence of diagnosed psoriasis is 3.15%. The prevalence in Africa varies depending on geographic location, being lowest in West Africa. Psoriasis is less prevalent in China [4] and Japan than in Europe, and has not been described in natives of the Andean region of South America [5, 6].

There are fewer reports on the incidence of psoriasis, but a study from Rochester, Minnesota, USA showed an increasing trend over the last 2 decades. The prevalence of PsA also shows similar variation, being highest in people of European descent and lowest in the Japanese. Although, study methodology and case definition may explain some of the variations, genetic and environmental factors are important [7].Genetic epidemiologic studies have shown that both diseases have a strong genetic component. Environmental risk factors including streptococcal pharyngitis, stressful life events, low humidity, drugs, HIV infection, trauma, smoking and obesity have been associated with psoriasis and PsA [8].

The genes involved, in PsA are HLA genes of class I major histocompatibility (MHC) alleles, on the HLA-B and HLA-C loci. Psoriasis is linked to HLA-Cw6 allele. Twenty percent of PsA patients with peripheral joint involvement displayed HLA-B27, a value that climbs to 70% in patients with PsA type spine involvement [9]. The overlap in associated HLA antigens for both diseases (B13, B17, B57, Cw6, and DR7) suggests a shared genetic predisposition [10].

Psoriasis and PsA are heritable diseases. Polymorphisms in the genes encoded in the MHC region have consistently been associated with psoriasis and PsA and account for about 30% of the genetic risk. In psoriasis, the association has been primarily with class I antigens: HLA-B13, HLA-B17, HLA-Cw6, and HLA-Cw7, the strongest association being with HLA-Cw6. Typing for HLA-Cw6 may have potential clinical utility, as it is associated with early onset of psoriasis, higher incidence of guttate or streptococcal induced disease flares, and more severe disease. PsA is also associated with multiple HLA antigens, many of which are similar to psoriasis antigens, as the two diseases are interrelated [11]. However, specific associations do exist for the inflammatory arthritis, as HLA-B27 is associated with greater spinal involvement, and B38 and B39 with peripheral polyarthritis. HLA antigens are also prognostic factors, as HLA-B39 alone, HLA-B27 in the presence of HLA-DR7, and HLA-DQw3 in the absence of HLA-DR7 all confer an increased risk for disease progression. The RA shared epitope was found to be associated with radiologic erosions among patients with PsA. Patients with PsA carrying both HLACw6 and HLA-DRB107 alleles were determined to have a less severe course of arthritis. Recently, the results of multiple well powered genome-wide association studies have identified several loci outside the MHC region associated with psoriasis risk, including three genes involved in interleukin (IL)-23 signaling (IL-23R, IL-23A, IL-12B), two genes that regulate nuclear factor-κB signaling (TNIP1, TNFAIP3), and two genes involved in the modulation of T-helper type 2 immune responses (IL-4, IL-13) [12].

For many years the concept of PsA as a separate disease entity was controversial, its importance has been underestimated. Dermatologists focus on psoriatic skin may overlook PsA due to its clinical heterogeneity or when only minor symptoms are present such as mild enthesitis or arthritis of DIP joints. Because skin lesions occur years before the manifestation of arthritis, however, it is likely that many patients are being seen by a dermatologist when PsA initially develops. A study among 1511 patients found 20% had PsA; in 85% of the cases PsA was newly diagnosed. Of these patients more than 95% had active arthritis and 53% had five or more joints affected. Polyarthritis (58%) was the most common manifestation pattern, followed by oligoarthritis (31%) and arthritis mutilans (4%). DIP involvement was present in 41% and dactylitis in 23% of the patients. Compared with patients without arthritis, patients with PsA had more severe skin symptoms (mean PASI 14.3 vs. 11.5), a lower quality of life and greater impairment of productivity parameters [13].

The CASPAR study group was established for classification criteria for PsA. The CASPAR criteria comprised: 1- Evidence of psoriasis (a) Current psoriatic skin or scalp disease present today as judged by a rheumatologist or dermatologist (b) Personal history of psoriasis that may be obtained from patient (c) Family history of psoriasis in a first or second degree relative according to patient report, family doctor, dermatologist, rheumatologist or other qualified health-care provider. 2- Psoriatic nail dystrophy including onycholysis, pitting and hyperkeratosis observed on current physical examination. 3- A negative test for rheumatoid factor by any method except latex but preferably by ELISA or nephelometry. 4- Dactylitis: a) current swelling of an entire digit b) history of dactylitis recorded by a rheumatologist. 5- Radiological evidence of juxta-articular new bone formation as ill-defined ossification near joint margins (but excluding osteophyte formation) on plain x rays of hand or foot. Using the CASPAR criteria, the combination of psoriasis and inflammatory arthritis gave 0.96 for sensitivity and 0.97 for specificity, respectively [14, 15, 16]. The Toronto group evaluated the use of the CASPAR criteria in early disease and found a sensitivity of 99.1% in those patients with disease duration of less than 2.5 years and a sensitivity of 100% for those with disease duration of less than 12 months [17].

Both dactylitis and enthesitis are hallmark features of PsA, and dactylitis is a severity marker for the disease. Spinal disease in PsA is qualitatively and quantitatively different from classical ankylosing spondylitis (AS), and a new scoring system combines elements of the "Bath Ankylosing Spondylitis Radiology Index" (BASRI) and "Modified Stoke AS Spinal Score" (mSASSS) to give a new modified index useful for definition of PsA types [18, 19].

The concept of spondyloarthritides (SpA) that comprised a group of interrelated disorders has been recognized since the early 1970s. The CASPAR study led to a new set of validated classification criteria for PsA and is widely used in clinical studies. In AS, the 1984 modified New York criteria have been used widely in clinical studies and daily practice but are not applicable in early disease when the characteristic radiographic signs of sacroiliitis are not visible but active sacroiliitis is readily detectable by magnetic resonance imaging (MRI). This led to the concept of axial SpA that includes patients with and without radiographic damage. Candidate criteria for axial SpA were developed based on proposals for a structured diagnostic approach. These criteria were validated in the "Assessment of Spondyloarthritis International Society" (ASAS) study on new classification criteria for axial SpA, a large international prospective study. In these new criteria, sacroiliitis showing up on MRI has been given as much weight as sacroiliitis on radiographs, thereby also identifying patients with early axial SpA. Both the CASPAR and the ASAS criteria for axial SpA are likely to be of use as diagnostic criteria to define PsA types [20].

Early PsA is a condition with a consistent risk of clinical progression. Abundant entheseal involvement is a distinctive clinical aspect that helps discriminate early PsA from RA. Today its detection, followed by a rapid therapeutic intervention, predicts a better clinical outcome [21]. Different to RA, the joint distribution in PsA tends to be asymmetrical and oligoarticular (< five joints). Distal joints, particularly the DIP joints of the hands, are more frequently affected; joint tenderness tends to be less; and dactylitis, enthesitis and axial or spinal involvement are more frequent. Unlike seronegative spondyloarthropathy, 40% of patients with PsA suffer from a sacroiliitis that tends to exhibit an asymmetrical rather than a symmetrical distribution. Other features of PsA include the absence of rheumatoid nodules, of rheumatoid factor in the blood and, in some instances, the presence of iritis, mucous membrane lesions, urethritis, bowel inflammation and tendonitis. PsA is often characterized by plain film evidence of juxta-articular new bone formation and magnetic resonance imaging evidence of enthesitis. Eighty per cent of cases are associated with psoriatic nail changes such as pitting, ridging, oil spots and nail plate thickening. Although PsA is preceded by cutaneous psoriasis in 75% of cases, in 10–15% of cases the arthritis precedes the psoriasis, suggesting that the two diseases may be controlled by different mechanisms or that a common etiology, may remains dormant in the synovial compartment. The mean time to onset of arthritis among those with pre-existing cutaneous psoriasis is 10 years, but delays have been reported of up to 20 years. Few instances of PsA without psoriasis have been described because most cases resembling PsA in the absence of personal or family history of skin disease are classified as an undifferentiated spondyloarthropathy [22, 23]. Patients with clinical symptoms and signs of PsA and a family history of psoriasis can be classified as having PsA *sine* psoriasis. The clinical spectrum of PsA *sine* psoriasis is broad. It is identified by dactylitis and/or DIP arthritis, HLA-Cw6, and a family history of psoriasis following the CASPAR criteria [24].

Psoriatic disease encompassing skin, joint and nail involvement is an autoimmune process as evidenced from animal models, the human leukocyte antigen (HLA)-Cw6 association in man, T cells infiltration in lesional skin and the response to T cell targeted therapies. The nails and joints are associated with inflammation at points of ligament or tendon insertion (i.e., enthesitis). It has been postulated that response to tissue stressing of the integrated nail-joint apparatus, rather than autoimmunity, is driving the inflammatory process with a relative differential involvement of adaptive and innate immunity in the psoriatic disease [25]. Nail fold psoriasis and DIP joint arthritis were associated with nail involvement and were common in PsA patients. Nail psoriasis has been postulated to be related to the Koebner phenomenon and local inflammatory DIP joint arthritis, and probably indicative of distal phalanx enthesitis in PsA patients [26]

A key objective of the assessment working group of the "Group for Research and Assessment of Psoriasis and Psoriatic Arthritis" (GRAPPA) was to identify, develop, evaluate, and validate outcome measures for use in clinical trials of PsA and in clinical practice useful in defining PsA types [27].

Biomarkers are helpful in screening patients with psoriasis for PsA types. Patients with psoriasis satisfying CASPAR criteria for PsA were analyzed for IL-12, IL-12p40, IL-17, TNF super family members (TNFSF14), MMP-3, RANK ligand (RANKL), osteoprotegerin (OPG), cartilage oligomeric matrix protein (COMP), C-propeptide of Type II collagen (CPII), collagen fragment neoepitopes Col2-3/4 long mono (C2C), Col2-3/4short (C1-2C) and highly sensitive CRP (hsCRP). Serum levels of RANKL, TNFSF14, MMP-3 and COMP independently associated with psoriatic disease. Twenty six PsA patients (mean swollen and tender joint count: 16, swollen joint count: 5) were then compared with 26 patients who had psoriasis alone. Increased levels of hsCRP, OPG, MMP-3 and the CPII:C2C ratios were independently associated with PsA and are biomarkers for PsA in patients with psoriasis [28].

Psoriatic Arthritis Health Effects

Epidemiological studies have shown that, in patients with psoriasis, associated disorders may occur more frequently than expected. Such comorbidities include PsA, inflammatory bowel disease, obesity, diabetes, and CVD, several cancer types, and depression. Comorbidities often become clinically manifest years after onset of psoriasis and tend to be more frequently seen in severe disease [29]. In particular, nonalcoholic fatty liver disease affects about 50%, Crohn's disease 0.5% and celiac disease 0.2 - 4.3% of patients with psoriasis. The presence of comorbidities has important implications in the global approach to patients. In particular, traditional systemic antipsoriatic agents could negatively affect cardio-metabolic comorbidities as well as nonalcoholic fatty liver disease and may have important interactions with drugs commonly used by psoriasis patients. Moreover, patients with psoriasis should be encouraged to drastically correct their modifiable cardiovascular and liver risk factors, in particular obesity, alcohol consumption, and smoking habit, because this could positively affect psoriasis, PsA and their life expectance [30].

A contributing role of nerve growth factor (NGF) mediated neuroimmunologic mechanisms has provided a new dimension in the understanding of various cutaneous and systemic inflammatory diseases and comorbidities. Recent evidence implicates NGF as a key mediator of inflammation and pain. NGF influences an inflammatory reaction by regulating neuropeptides, angiogenesis, cell trafficking molecules, and T cell activation. The recognition of a pathologic role of NGF and its receptor system has provided an attractive opportunity to develop a novel class of therapeutics for inflammatory diseases and chronic pain syndromes [31].

Clinical measures of disease activity were related to fatigue over time; however, these relationships disappeared in the context of patient reported physical disability and pain. Patient reported measures of physical disability, pain, and psychological distress were most closely related to higher "Modified Fatigue Severity Scale" (mFSS) scores (greater fatigue) across clinic assessments. Fatigue was found to vary over time, at least when assessed at yearly intervals. In general, measures of clinical and functional status at the current visit were more predictive of change in mFSS scores in between previous and current visits than change scores between visits. Comorbid fibromyalgia and hypertension were also associated with greater fatigue across multiple visits and with change in fatigue between visits. A combination of factors is associated with fatigue in PsA [32].

The number of actively inflamed joints as measure of disease activity and the number of clinically deformed joints as measure of damage were significantly related to the "Health Assessment Questionnaire" (HAQ) score also useful for defining PsA types. Furthermore, interaction terms for illness duration with the number of actively inflamed joints were statistically significant, with or without inclusion of the erythrocyte sedimentation rate and morning stiffness in the model. The influence of disease activity on HAQ scores declines with increased disease duration [33].

The prevalence of obesity in psoriatic patients within the "Utah Psoriasis Initiative" (UPI) population was higher than that in the general Utah population. Obesity appears to be the consequence of psoriasis and not a risk factor for onset of disease. It was not observed an increased risk for PsA in patients with obesity; furthermore, obesity did not affect the response or adverse effects of topical corticosteroids, light based treatments, and systemic medications. The prevalence of smoking in the UPI population was higher than in the general Utah population and higher than in the non-psoriatic population. It was found a higher prevalence of smokers in the obese population within the UPI than in the obese population within the Utah population [34].

In a population of patients with PsA 23.3% had renal abnormalities as defined by creatinine clearance below the lower cut off of normal distribution and urinary excretion of albumin more than 25 mg/24 hrs. These patients were significantly older at the time of the study, older at joint disease onset, had longer skin disease duration, increased serum levels of beta2-microglobulin, and higher incidence of increased erythrocyte sedimentation rate and C reactive protein levels [35].

Patients with PsA have an increased incidence of CVD and cardiovascular risk factors such as smoking, hypertension, and metabolic syndrome compared to the normal population as well as nonconventional risk factors such as raised levels of homocysteine and excessive alcohol consumption. In patients with PsA, carotid wave pulse velocity, a measure of arterial stiffness, was significantly higher. Patients with psoriasis were found to have increased coronary artery calcification in direct imaging study compared to controls. Two case control studies also demonstrated that patients with PsA had a higher prevalence of subclinical atherosclerosis as measured by arterial IMT and endothelial dysfunction without overt CVD. In patients without clinical CVD 35% had increased IMT despite having low cardiovascular risk. Patients with PsA had a higher prevalence ratio for type II diabetes, hyperlipidemia, and hypertension compared to controls. One hundred two patients with PsA had a higher prevalence of diabetes mellitus and hypertension, and an increased prevalence of HDL cholesterol, apolipoprotein A1 levels, lower total cholesterol and LDL cholesterol levels, and lower total cholesterol to HDL cholesterol ratio. Chronic inflammation has been shown to play a role in the development of atherosclerosis now considered as an inflammatory, autoimmune like disease. Both the innate immune system and T helper-1 lymphocytes appear to be involved in atherogenesis. This is similar to the pattern of immune mediated inflammation in psoriasis and PsA. It is possible that psoriasis and PsA produce chronic, systemic inflammation, with higher levels of inflammatory cells and cytokines invoking endothelial inflammation and plaque formation in the vascular system [36].

The event rates and rate ratios (RRs) of cardiovascular death, myocardial infarct (MI), coronary revascularization, stroke and a composite of MI, stroke and cardiovascular death were increased in patients with psoriasis. The RRs increased with disease severity and decreased with age of onset. The risk was similar in patients with severe skin affection alone and those with PsA [37].

The increased risk for CVD in RA is well known and inflammation appears to play a pivotal etiological role. There is now substantial interest in whether or not PsA is also associated with an enhanced cardiovascular risk. In all patients CVD was defined as a history of MI, stroke and/or transient ischemic attack verified by written documentation of the event. The prevalence of CVD was 10% in patients with PsA compared with 12% in patients with RA [38].

Several studies provide support for augmented cardiovascular risk, represented by both functional and structural arterial wall changes in PsA. Flow-mediated dilatation (FMD) was significantly impaired in PsA patients without traditional cardiovascular risk factors or CVD compared with matched controls. Another study also showed a higher prevalence of subclinical atherosclerosis, as measured by carotid IMT, among PsA patients. As in RA, CVD and their risk factors including hyperlipidaemia, diabetes mellitus and hypertension were more common in PsA patients than in matched controls [39]. However, mortality in patients with PsA, in a single center cohort was not significantly different from the general population in England. No increased risk of death was observed in this cohort [40].

To evaluate the prevalence of the metabolic syndrome (MetS), patients with RA, AS and PsA were recruited for a study of atherosclerotic risk factors and the MetS, defined according to the 2009 Joint Statements using the Asian criteria for central obesity. The prevalence of MetS was significantly higher in PsA (38%) than RA (20%) or AS (11%). Patients with PsA had significantly higher prevalence of impaired fasting glucose (30%), low HDL-cholesterol (33%), high triglyceride (21%), central obesity (65%) and high blood pressure (56%). Patients with PsA, but not RA or AS, have a significantly higher prevalence of the MetS syndrome compared to the general population. Among the three diseases studied, PsA has the highest prevalence of the MetS and is associated with highest cardiovascular risk [41, 42].

A cohort analysis of PsA patients who were followed up prospectively from 1978 to 2004 at the University of Toronto PsA Clinic was performed. Of the 665 patients included, 68 (10.2%) developed a malignancy at an average age of 62.4 years. The most frequently seen malignancies were breast (20.6%), lung (13.2%), and prostate (8.8%) cancer. However, the incidence of malignancy in the large PsA cohort did not differ from that in the general population [43].

Psoriatic Arthritis Therapies

Psoriasis is one of the most prevalent chronic inflammatory diseases with a high economic impact. The disease persists for life, and the patient has an increased risk of CVD. One out of five patients develops PsA. The clinical picture of psoriasis is highly variable with regard to lesion characteristics and the severity of disease. To improve the management of psoriasis, guidelines must be followed and all appropriate topical and systemic treatment options must be tried, with clearly defined treatment goals. The spectrum of established systemic treatments for psoriasis has been extended by the biologics [44].

PsA is an inflammatory arthritis occurring in up to 30% of patients with psoriasis. Its clear distinction from RA has been described clinically, genetically, and immunohistologically. Therapies that target cells, such as activated T cells, proinflammatory cytokines, and TNFα, are used extensively today. A variety of items are evaluated including joints, skin, enthesium, dactylitis, spine function, quality of life, and imaging assessment of disease activity and damage[45]. The performance of treatments in these various domains have being evaluated by GRAPPA, and improved measures are being developed and validated specifically for PsA. Traditional therapies for PsA like NSAIDs, oral immunomodulatory drugs, topical creams, and light therapy have been helpful in controlling both musculoskeletal and dermatologic lesions of the disease, but may eventually show diminished benefit, and may produce severe toxicities as side effects [46]. The primary goals in the treatment of PsA are reduction of pain; improvement in the other signs and symptoms of disease, including skin and nail involvement; optimization of functional capacity and quality of life; and inhibition of the progression of joint damage. These goals should be achieved while minimizing potential toxicities from treatment. The management of PsA should simultaneously target arthritis, skin disease, and other manifestations of PsA, including involvement of the axial skeleton dactylitis, enthesitis, and eye inflammation. In this respect targeted biological agents, primarily TNFα inhibitors, have emerged as generally well tolerated and highly effective alternatives to traditional "Disease Modifying Anti Rheumatic Drugs" (DMARDs) [47]

PsA was considered as a less damaging disease than RA. In early arthritis 50% of patients showed significant joint damage developing erosions in the first 2 years even if DMARDs were used as treatment [3]. The treatment should aim to preserve function, prevent disability and maintain quality of life. The therapeutic approach has employed treatments to benefit both the skin and joints with minimal adverse effects, and to prevent subsequent disability and damage, inflammation i.e. synovitis which must be arrested and controlled early. In this respect combination therapy with conventional DMARDs and biologic drugs, like TNFα inhibitors, has made significant progress in the last 10 years. A remission rate of 58% of patients treated with DMARD and biologic therapy for 12 months has been achieved [48].

Nail involvement in psoriasis is typically overlooked; it can affect up to 50% of patients with psoriasis and cause functional impact as well as psychological stress that affect quality of life. Psoriatic patients with nail disease have more severe skin lesions, and higher rate of unremitting PsA. The current management of nail psoriasis includes topical, intralesional and systemic therapies, although little clinical evidence is available on the effectiveness of conventional treatments. Biologic agents are beginning to emerge as a viable option to treat patients with both cutaneous and nail clinical manifestations of psoriasis and PsA [49].

Although they can have some beneficial effect on skin disease and peripheral arthritis, there is lack of evidence for DMARDs, such as methotrexate (MTX), Leflunomide (LEF), cyclosporine (CsA), and sulfasalazine (SSZ) in affecting dactylitis or enthesitis, and they are clearly ineffective in axial disease. Systemic glucocorticoids may cause a flare of psoriasis if tapered too quickly, and should be used with caution in PsA. In contrast, biologics, particularly TNFα inhibitors seem to be beneficial in skin psoriasis and across of all the manifestations of PsA, including arthritis, skin and nail disease, spinal disease, enthesitis and dactylitis. They also improve quality of life and inhibit joint damage. All the currently used TNFα inhibitors appear to have comparable efficacy and safety profiles in patients with PsA. They can be used as monotherapy or in combination with MTX or other traditional DMARDs. Initiation of anti-TNFα agents is recommended for patients who failed one of the traditional DMARDs or as an initial therapy in patients who have poor prognosis. Other biological agents, including alefacept and abatacept, appear to be less potent than TNFα inhibitors in PsA and their use is likely to be reserved for patients who failed or cannot be treated with TNFα inhibitors. These agents are usually used in combination with other DMARDs. The Efficacy of ustekinumab in the treatment of PsA has been recently reported and is presently under further investigation [45, 48, 49, 50, 51].

Results from clinical trials of biologic anti-TNFα drugs confirmed the biological relevance of TNFα function in the pathogenesis of chronic noninfectious inflammation of joints, skin and gut. Up to April 2009, more than two million patients worldwide have received the first marketed drugs, namely the monoclonal anti-TNFα antibodies infliximab and adalimumab and the soluble TNF receptor etanercept. All three are equally effective in RA, AS, psoriasis and PsA, and only the monoclonal antibodies are effective in inflammatory bowel disease. The spectrum of efficacy with anti-TNFα therapies includes diseases such as systemic vasculitis and sight-threatening uveitis. New adverse effects are recognized, like development of new onset psoriasis, reactivation of latent tuberculosis remains the most important safety issue of anti-TNFα therapies [52].

RA, AS and PsA are commonly thought of as inflammatory diseases that affect younger individuals. The safety profiles for etanercept, infliximab and adalimumab in patients of 65 years or more, anti-TNFα treatments for an active inflammatory disease such as RA, AS or PsA, or psoriasis were analyzed. Anti TNFα treatment is a safe option possibly leading to better disease outcome [53].

Altogether there is sufficient reason not to dismiss traditional agents for use in PsA because of lack of evidence. Also, due consideration must be given to the considerable cost of biologic treatments versus traditional treatments. The role of combination therapy with TNFα inhibitors is an important one, especially considering that 30%–40% of patients in the TNFα inhibitor trials have been on MTX as concomitant medication [54].

Traditional systemic therapies for psoriasis, such as MTX, CsA, retinoids or psoralen plus ultraviolet light (PUVA) therapy, have a potential for long-term toxicity and may not always provide sufficient improvement of the disease. Biological therapies for the treatment of PsA are defined by their mode of action and can be classified into three categories: the T-cell modulating agents (alefacept and efalizumab), the TNFα blockers, (adalimumab, certolizumab, etanercept, golimumab and infliximab) and the inhibitors of interleukin IL-12 and IL-23 (ustekinumab and briakinumab) [55].

DMARDs remain the first choice for the treatment of peripheral arthritis despite scarce evidence of their efficacy or ability to halt radiographic progression. TNFα antagonists have the greatest level of evidence for symptom control and radiographic progression. They are currently used after the failure of DMARDs to effectively treat peripheral arthritis, enthesitis, and dactylitis, and are the first choice when axial disease predominates. Despite the use of these treatments, 30% to 40% of patients will still have active disease. Among new drugs, evidence of efficacy has already been published with regard to anti-IL12/23 monoclonal antibody (ustekimumab) and golimumab [56].

For a long time, the endothelial covering of the vessels has been considered an inert surface. On the contrary, the endothelial cells are active and dynamic elements in the interaction between blood and tissues. The control of the vessel basal tone is obtained by the complex balance between the relaxing and contracting endothelial factors. Previous clinical studies show that patients suffering from RA and other autoimmune rheumatologic pathologies are at high risk of death being prematurely affected by atherosclerosis and CVD. Blocking TNFα by biological drugs improves the endothelial function. The effects of two anti-TNFα drugs (infliximab and etanercept) on the endothelial function were evaluated by FMD, which was measured in the brachial artery before and after treatment. 36 patients were enrolled 25 with RA and 11 with PsA. They were divided into three groups: 10 patients were treated with etanercept, 13 with infliximab, and 13 with DMARDs. The carotid IMT was measured and the endothelial function was evaluated by FMD measurement in the brachial artery, before treatment, 1 h after the beginning of treatment and after 8–12 weeks. No statistically significant difference between the three groups before treatment was found for the ultrasonographic evaluation of the carotid IMT. On the contrary, the differences between FMD values before and after the treatment in the patients treated with etanercept and in the patients treated with infliximab were statistically significant. Long-term evaluation for infliximab and etanercept was performed by comparing the FMD values, 8 and 12 weeks after the first treatment. After 8 weeks, FMD value was similar to the value recorded at enrollment in the infliximab group and the FMD values in the etanercept group after 12 weeks showed a not statistically significant reduction of vasodilatating effect. Drugs in patients affected by autoimmune arthritis can modify the endothelial function, as indicated by the induced FMD changes, but the long-term effect tends to be considerably reduced [57].

Significantly diminished values for swollen and tender joints, patients global and pain assessments, doctor's global assessment of disease activity, erythrocyte sedimentation rate, C-reactive protein, and "Health Assessment Questionnaire" (HAQ) score were observed within 3 months after commencement of both infliximab and etanercept. Values remained significantly lower throughout the 24 months of follow up. ACR20 response at 3 months was 79% (n = 22/28) for infliximab and 76% (n = 34/45) for etanercept. The first biological drug was discontinued in 16% due to lack of effectiveness and in 6% due to adverse events [58].

It is unclear if skin cancer risk is affected by the use of immunomodulatory medications in RA, psoriasis, and PsA. RA may potentiate the risk of cutaneous malignancy and therefore dermatologic screening in this population should be considered. The use of immunomodulatory therapy in RA, psoriasis, and PsA may further increase the risk of cutaneous malignancy and therefore dermatologic screening examinations are warranted in these groups. More careful recording of skin cancer development during clinical trials and cohort studies is necessary to further delineate the risks of immunomodulatory therapy [59].

PsA provides an ideal disease model in which to investigate the bioactivities of potentially therapeutic cytokines at multiple sites of tissue inflammation. The effects of subcutaneous rhIL-10, an anti-inflammatory cytokine, was investigated for 28 days in a double-blind, placebo-controlled study in PsA patients. Synovial/skin biopsies, peripheral blood leukocytes, articular magnetic resonance images, and clinical disease activity scores were obtained sequentially. Modest, but significant clinical improvement in skin, but not articular disease activity scores with only minor adverse effects was observed. Type 1, but not Type 2 cytokine production in vitro was suppressed in human rhIL-10 treatment compared with placebo recipients. Similarly, TNFα and IL-1β, production in whole blood stimulated with LPS in vitro was reduced, whereas serum soluble TNFRII levels were elevated, indicating suppression of monocyte function. Decreased T cell and macrophage infiltration in synovial tissues was accompanied by reduced P-selectin expression. Moreover, suppressed synovial enhancement on magnetic resonance imaging and reduced alpha(v)beta(3) integrin expression on von Willebrand factor(+) vessels were observed. Together these data demonstrate that a short course of IL-10 modulates immune responses in vivo via diverse effects on endothelial activation, leukocyte recruitment and effector functions. Such biological changes may result in clinically meaningful improvement in disease activity [60].

Biologic agents should be considered for use solely in children with psoriasis that is refractory to conventional therapies, including children with severe, widespread, refractory pustular, plaque or PsA. Etanercept appears to have resulted in less severe side effects compared to infliximab in the juvenile RA population. Serious adverse events (including infection), have been reported in the literature and should be taken into account before beginning treatment with any biologic agent [61].

The socioeconomic scenario of PsA is similar to RA. Current treatments do not achieve remission of symptoms or prevention of the appearance of damage in the early stage of PsA nor the blocking of PsA progression in old cases. The current management of PsA includes NSAIDs, corticosteroids, DMARDs and anti-TNF-α alpha blocking agents. These biologic drugs are more effective than traditional DMARDs on inflammation, quality of life and function and can inhibit the progression of the structural joint damage. Recent advancement in the immunopathogenesis of PsA has permitted the development of novel drugs including new TNF-α blockers, IL-1, IL-6, IL-12, IL-23 and IL-17 inhibitors, co-stimulator modulation inhibitors, B-cell depleting agents, small molecules and receptor activator of NF-kappaB/receptor activator of NF-kappaB ligand inhibitors [62].

Baseline clinical characteristics including demographics, previous DMARDs response, tender and swollen joint counts, early morning stiffness, pain visual analogue score, patient global assessment, C reactive protein (CRP) and HAQ were collected. At 12 months remission, defined according to the disease activity score using 28 joint count and CRP (DAS28-CRP), was achieved in 58% of PsA patients compared to 44% of RA patients. DAS28 remission is possible in PsA patients at one year following anti-TNFα therapy, at higher rates than in RA patients and is predicted by baseline HAQ [63].

Therapy for inflammatory joint diseases, such as RA, AS and PsA, includes DMARDs. Conventional DMARDs are used as monotherapy or in combination and include MTX, LEF, azathioprine, CsA, hydroxychloroquine, SSZ, gold and minocycline. Biologic therapies are TNFα inhibitors, T-cell modulators and B-cell depleters. They have all been shown to have clinical efficacy and are able to retard structural damage [64].

While treating subjects in Venezuela with a vaccine containing *Leishmania* amastigotes antigens for prevention of cutaneous leishmaniasis (CL), we observed 100% clinical remission of a psoriatic lesion in one subject, a natural double blind serendipity finding. A first generation polyvalent vaccine (AS100-1) was manufactured with protein from four cultured *Leishmania* species. A double-blind, placebo-controlled, parallel group study, of multiple doses of AS100-1 was performed on psoriatic subjects, to confirm safety and efficacy [65]. Treatment of plaque psoriasis, was conducted in 2,770 volunteers and included plaque (79%), guttate (10%), plaque and guttate (10%), palm/plantar (0.3%), erythrodermia (1.8%), inverse (0.8%), plaque and arthritis (3.4%) and nail psoriasis (0.3%). Baseline PASI compared with post-treatment values were: PASI 100, 23%; PASI 75, 45%; PASI 50, 13%; PASI 10, 9%; <PASI 10, 3% while 7% quit treatment. There were no serious

adverse events attributed to the treatment drug. Some patients with PsA benefited after treatment [65]. To determine the effective factor, a single blind trial with four monovalent second generation vaccines (AS100-2) was performed in 26 subjects, which also had remission of psoriasis. AS100-2 vaccines were further purified, resulting in seven chromatography fractions (AS200) per species. Subsequently, a single-blind trial in 55 subjects treated with a third generation vaccine AS200 prepared with DEAE chromatography fractions from L(V)brasiliensis also induced remission of psoriasis. Interestingly, two HIV+ subjects with plaque psoriasis experienced remission after treatment with AS100-1 [66]. AS200 Leishmania antigenic fractions induced linear delayed type hypersensitivity (DTH) reactions in guinea pigs over a 1-40 µg dose range. This finding allowed us to build a potency assay for the drug product. Furthermore AS200 fractions also induced remission of lesions in a mice collagen model for RA [67].

Peripheral blood mononuclear cells (PBMC) collected from subjects prior to treatment and post-treatment with AS100-1 were analyzed by flow cytometry. Upon analysis, it was noticed that lymphocyte subsets (LS) varied with PASI range (1-10, 11-20 and 21-72). Pretreatment absolute values of gated LS were as follows: CD4+CD8-, CD3+CD8-, CD8+CD3+, CD8+CD4- and CD8+HLA- decreased in PBMC as PASI increased, suggesting migration from the blood to the skin. Contrary to the previous finding, the following LS, CD8+HLA+, HLA+CD8-, CD8+CD4+, CD19, and membrane surface immunoglobulin IgA+, IgD+ and IgM+ increased in PBMC as PASI increased, suggesting activation and proliferation by unknown antigens in the skin lesions. After treatment with seven doses of AS100-1, the following LS, CD3+CD8-, CD8+CD3-, HLA+CD8-, CD8+HLA+ and CD4+CD8-, increased as PASI returns to normal values and psoriatic plaques disappeared, while CD8+CD3+, CD8+HLA-, CD19 and CD8+CD4+ decreased in PBMC suggesting lower sensitization in skin. Lymphocyte trafficking from blood to skin decreased significantly, stopping the vicious cycle as psoriasis lesions disappeared [68].

Inflammatory markers C-reactive protein (CRP) and complement 5a (C5a) assayed in PsA patients decreased significantly in serum after treatment with 6 doses of AS200 DEAE fractions 3 + 4 Leishmania amastigotes antigens. The Leishmania antigens decreased markedly the TNFα concentration in supernatants from PBMC in both patients and controls. In mice Concanavalin A (ConA) induced hepatitis, injection of AS100-2 L(L)chagasi antigens subcutaneously decreased serum TNFα compared with placebo in 8 hours of observation. Serum IL-1β, 8 hours after SC injection of AS200 and AS100-1 in mice also decreased significantly compared with placebo and in a range similar to the positive control dexamethasone. AS100-2 *L(L)chagasi* antigens decreased proliferation of cutaneous T cell lymphoma in vitro in a dose–response relationship [69].

As more skin disease is present in PsA patients, more inflammation is found in the joints, suggesting a link between skin and joint inflammatory processes; since both were exacerbated in the PASI 100 and PASI 75 groups and also needed higher number of doses to achieve a lower AS, tender joints and nail changes values. Gated Absolute values of gated LS before treatment decreased in this order: CD8+HLA-, CD8+HLA+, CD4+, CD8+CD3+, CD8+CD3 in PBMC as PASI increased, suggesting migration of CD8+ cells from the blood to the joints and skin. Contrary to the previous finding, LS: CD8+CD4-, CD3+CD8-, HLA+CD8-, CD19+, CD8+CD4+, IgA+, IgD+, IgM+, IgE+, and IgG+ increased in PBMC as PASI increased suggesting activation and proliferation by unknown antigens.

The LS quantification in this group of PsA patients only (n=508) were different to the LS quantified in the psoriasis skin disease trial (n=2770) [68], since in PsA the majority belonged to the CD8+ phenotype, a T cell key in the PsA inflammatory process as described by many authors. In PsA patients there is also evidence of T cell recirculation before treatment and a vicious cycle with T and B cells migrating between blood and skin and joints. After treatment with nine doses of AS100-1 *Leishmania* amastigotes antigens, a dramatic decrease in all T and B LS in PBMC was observed, as PASI, AS, tender joint counts, and nail changes returns to normal values and the vicious cycle disappeared [70]. AS100-1 had a cellular not humoral immune response as supported by the DTH and ELISA results in humans and guinea pigs [65-67]. All psoriatic patients were DTH positive after the third vaccination with AS100-1, but no ELISA antibodies were detected in serum from these volunteers up to 6 doses of vaccine [65].

This suggests that the immunological response to AS100-1 after TLCK treatment and NP-40 extraction was mediated by immunization of T-regulatory cells, with no antibody production, a novel mechanism that may play a role in decreasing inflammation in psoriatic skin. Amastigote peptides may induce Th3 regulatory T cells producing IL-10 that inhibits Th1 and Th2 cell cytokine production and induced peripheral cell tolerance.

CONCLUSION

TNFα decreased with amastigote antigens [69] and has been implicated in many diseases as Crohn's disease, multiple sclerosis, Alzheimer's disease, transplant rejection, type II diabetes, rheumatoid arthritis, heart failure, atherosclerosis, allergic asthma, liver disease, tumorigenesis, tumor metastasis, lymphoproliferative diseases, pulmonary fibrosis, and systemic lupus erythematosus, most of them with disease models in experimental animals that should be tested to analyze the effect of amastigote antigens in their potential regression for the benefit of human beings.

REFERENCES

[1] Gladman DD. (2009) Psoriatic Arthritis from Wright's Era until today. *J. Rheumatol.* 83: 4-8.

[2] Moll JM, Wright V (1973) Psoriatic arthritis. *Semin. Arthritis Rheum* 3(1):55–78.

[3] Gladman DD, Shuckett R, Russell ML, Thorne JC, Schachter RK (1987) Psoriatic arthritis (PSA)—an analysis of 220 patients. *Q. J. Med.* 62:127–141.

[4] Leung YY, Tam LS, Ho KW, Lau WN, Li TK, Zhu TY, Kun EW, Li EK. (2010) Evaluation of the CASPAR criteria for psoriatic arthritis in the Chinese population. *Rheumatology* 49:112–115.

[5] Chandran V, Raychaudhuri SP (2010) Geoepidemiology and environmental factors of psoriasis and psoriatic arthritis. *J. Autoimmun* 34:314-321.

[6] Chang YT, Chen TJ, Liu PC et al (2009) Epidemiological study of psoriasis in the national health insurance database in Taiwan. *Acta Derm Venereol.* 89:262-266.

[7] Gabriel SE, Michaud K (2009) Epidemiological studies in incidence, prevalence, mortality, and comorbidity of the rheumatic diseases. *Arthritis Res. Ther* 11:229-245.

[8]   Cantini F, Niccoli L, Nannini C, Kaloudi O, Bertoni M, Cassara E. Psoriatic arthritis: a systematic review. International Journal of *Rheumatic Diseases* 2010; 13: 300–317.

[9]   Amherd-Hoekstra A, Näher H, Lorenz HM et al (2010) Psoriatic arthritis: a review. *J. Dutsch Dermatol.Ges.* 8:332-339.

[10] Barton AC (2002) Genetic epidemiology. Psoriatic arthritis. *Arthritis Res* 4:247-251.

[11] O'Rielly DD, Rahman P (2010) Where Do We Stand With the Genetics of Psoriatic Arthritis? *Curr. Rheumatol Rep.* 12:300–308.

[12] Bowes J, Barton A. (2010). The genetics of psoriatic arthritis: lessons from genome-wide association studies. *Discov. Med.* 10:177-183.

[13] Reich K, Krüger K, Mössner R, Augustin M. (2009) Epidemiology and clinical pattern of psoriatic arthritis in Germany: a prospective interdisciplinary epidemiological study of 1511 patients with plaque-type psoriasis. *Br. J. Dermatol.* 160:1040–1047.

[14] Taylor W, Gladman D, Helliwell P, Marchesoni A, Mease P, Mielants H (2006) Classification criteria for psoriatic arthritis: development of new criteria from a large international study. *Arthritis Rheum* 54:2665–2673.

[15] Chandran V, Schentag CT, Gladman DD (2007) Sensitivity of the classification of psoriatic arthritis criteria in early psoriatic arthritis. *Arthritis Rheum* 57:1560-1563.

[16] Coates LC, Helliwell PS. (2008) Classification and categorization of psoriatic arthritis. *Clin. Rheumatol.* 27:1211-1216.

[17] Chandran V, Schentag CT, Gladman DD (2007) Sensitivity of the classification of psoriatic arthritis criteria in early psoriatic arthritis. *Arthritis Rheum.* 57:1560–1563.

[18] Helliwell PS (2009) Established Psoriatic Arthritis: *Clinical Aspects. J. Rheumatol.* 83:21-23.

[19] Coates LC, Helliwell PS. (2010) Disease measurement--enthesitis, skin, nails, spine and dactylitis. *Best Pract Res Clin. Rheumatol.* 24:659-70.

[20] Rudwaleit M, Taylor WJ. (2010) Classification criteria for psoriatic arthritis and ankylosing spondylitis/axial spondyloarthritis. 24:589-604.

[21] Scarpa R, Atteno M, Costa L, Peluso R, Iervolino S, Caso F, Del Puente A. (2009) Early psoriatic arthritis. *J. Rheumatol.* 83 26-27.

[22] Ciocon DH, Kimball AB (2007) Psoriasis and psoriatic arthritis: separate or one and the same? *Br. J. Dermatol.* 157: 850–860.

[23] Garg A, Gladman D (2010) Recognizing psoriatic arthritis in the dermatology clinic. *J. Am. Acad. Dermatol.* 63:733-748.

[24] Olivieri I, Padula A, D'Angelo S, Cutro MS. (2009) Psoriatic arthritis sine psoriasis. *J. Rheumatol.* 83:28-29.

[25] McGonagle D, Palmou Fontana N, Tan AL, Benjamin M. (2010) Nailing down the genetic and immunological basis for psoriatic Dermatology 221 (Suppl. 1):15-22 (DOI: 10.1159/000316171).

[26] Maejima H, Taniguchi T, Watarai A, Katsuoka K. (2010) Evaluation of nail disease in psoriatic arthritis by using a modified nail psoriasis severity score index. *Int. J. Dermatol.* 49:901-6.

[27] Mease PJ. Assessment tools in psoriatic arthritis. *J. Rheumatol.* (2008) 35:1426-30.

[28] Chandran V, Cook RJ, Edwin J, Shen H, Pellett FJ, Shanmugarajah S, Rosen CF, Gladman DD (2010). Soluble biomarkers differentiate patients with psoriatic arthritis from those with psoriasis without arthritis. *Rheumatology* 49:1399–1405.

[29] Naldi L, Mercuri SR. (2010) Epidemiology of comorbidities in psoriasis. *Dermatol. Ther.* 23(2):114-8.

[30] Gisondi P, Del Giglio M, Cozzi A. Girolomoni G. (2010) Psoriasis, the liver, and the gastrointestinal tract. *Dermatol. Ther* 23: 155–159.

[31] Raychaudhuri SK, Raychaudhuri SP. (2009) NGF and its receptor system: a new dimension in the pathogenesis of psoriasis and psoriatic arthritis. *Ann. N Y Acad. Sci.* 1173:470-477.

[32] Husted JA, Tom BD, Farewell VT, Gladman DD. (2010) Longitudinal analysis of fatigue in psoriatic arthritis. *J. Rheumatol.* 37:1878-1884.

[33] Husted JA, Tom BD, Farewell VT, Schentag CT, Gladman DD. (2007) A longitudinal study of the effect of disease activity and clinical damage on physical function over the course of psoriatic arthritis: Does the effect change over time? *Arthritis Rheum.* 56:840-849.

[34] Herron MD, Hinckley M, Hoffman MS, Papenfuss J, Hansen CB, Callis KP, Krueger GG. (2005) Impact of obesity and smoking on psoriasis presentation and management. *Arch. Dermatol.* 141:1527-1534.

[35] Alenius GM, Stegmayr BG, Dahlqvist SR. (2001). Renal abnormalities in a population of patients with psoriatic arthritis. *Scand. J. Rheumatol.* 30:271-274.

[36] Tobin AM, Veale DJ, Fitsgerald O, Rogers S, Collins P, O'Shea D, Kirby B (2010) Cardiovascular Disease and Risk Factors in Patients with Psoriasis and Psoriatic Arthritis. *J. Rheumatol.* 37:1386-1394.

[37] Ahlehoff O, Gislason GH, Charlot M, Jørgensen CH, Lindhardsen J, Olesen JB, Abildstrøm SZ, Skov L, Torp-Pedersen C, Hansen PR. (2010) Psoriasis is associated with clinically significant cardiovascular

risk: a Danish nationwide cohort study. *J. Intern. Med. doi:* 10.1111/j.1365-2796.2010.02310.x.

[38] Jamnitski A, Visman IM, Peters MJ, Boers M, Dijkmans BA, Nurmohamed MT. (2010) Prevalence of cardiovascular diseases in psoriatic arthritis resembles that of rheumatoid arthritis. Ann Rheum Dis. doi: 10.1136/ard.2010.136499.

[39] Bisoendial RJ, Stroes ES, Tak PP. (2009) Where the immune response meets the vessel wall. *Neth. J. Med.* 67:328-333.

[40] Buckley C, Cavill C, Taylor G, Kay H, Waldron N, Korendowych E, McHugh N. (2010) Mortality in psoriatic arthritis a single center study from the UK. *J. Rheumatol.* 37:2141-2144.

[41] Mok C, Ko G, Ho L, Yu K, Chan P, To C. (2010) Prevalence of atherosclerotic risk factors and the metabolic syndrome in patients with chronic inflammatory arthritis. Arthritis Care Res (Hoboken). DOI 10.1002/acr.20363

[42] Papo D, Hein R, Ring J. (2010) Psoriasis as an independent risk factor for development of coronary artery disease. *Dtsch Med Wochenschr.* 135:1749-54.

[43] Rohekar S, Tom BDM, Hassa A, Schentag CT, Farewell VT, Gladman DD. (2008) Prevalence of Malignancy in Psoriatic arthritis. *Arthritis and Rheumatism* 58:82–87.

[44] Mrowietz U, Reich K. (2009) Psoriasis--new insights into pathogenesis and treatment. *Dtsch Arztebl Int.* 106:11-18.

[45] Ceponis A, Kavanaugh A. (2010) Treatment of Psoriatic Arthritis with Biological Agents *Semin Cutan Med. Surg.* 29:56-62.

[46] Mease P. (2006) Psoriatic Arthritis Update. *Bull NYU Hosp. Jt Dis.* 64, Numbers 1 and 2.

[47] Mease PJ. (2010) Psoriatic Arthritis: Pharmacotherapy Update *Curr. Rheumatol. Rep.* 12:272–280.

[48] Wollina U, Unger L, Heinig B, Kittner T. (2010). Psoriatic arthritis. *Dermatol Ther.* 23:123–136.

[49] Vena GA, Vestita M, Cassano N (2010).Can early treatment with biologicals modify the natural history of comorbidities? *Dermatol. Ther.* 23:181–193.

[50] Mease PJ. (2010) Psoriatic arthritis - update on pathophysiology, assessment, and management. *Bull NYU Hosp Jt Dis.* 68:191-198.

[51] Mease PJ. Psoriatic arthritis assessment and treatment update. (2009) *Curr. Opin. Rheumatol.* 21:348-55.

[52] Sfikakis PP. (2010) The first decade of biologic TNF antagonists in clinical practice: lessons learned, unresolved issues and future directions. *Curr. Dir Autoimmun.* 11:180-210.

[53] Migliore A, Bizzi E, Laganà B, Altomonte L, Zaccari G, Granata M, Canzoni M, Marasini B, Massarotti M, Massafra U, Ranieri M, Pilla R, Martin LS, Pezza M, Vacca F, Galluccio A. (2009) The safety of anti-TNF agents in the elderly. *Int. J. Immunopathol Pharmacol.* 22:415-26.

[54] McHugh NJ. (2009) Traditional schemes for treatment of psoriatic arthritis. *J. Rheumatol.* 83:49-51.

[55] Weger W. (2010) Current status and new developments in the treatment of psoriasis and psoriatic arthritis with biological agents. *Br. J. Pharmacol.* 160:810-820.

[56] Soriano ER, Rosa J. (2009) Update on the treatment of peripheral arthritis in psoriatic arthritis. *Curr. Rheumatol. Rep.* 11:270-277.

[57] Mazzoccoli G, Notarsanto I, de Pinto GD, Dagostino MP, De Cata A, D'Alessandro G, Tarquini R, Vendemiale G. (2010) Anti-tumor necrosis factor-α therapy and changes of flow-mediated vasodilatation in psoriatic and rheumatoid arthritis patients. *Intern Emerg. Med.* 5:495-500.

[58] Virkki LM, Sumathikutty BC, Aarnio M, Valleala H, Heikkilä R, Kauppi M, Karstila K, Pirilä L, Ekman P, Salomaa S, Romu M, Seppälä J, Niinisalo H, Konttinen YT, Nordström DC. (2010) Biological therapy for psoriatic arthritis in clinical practice: outcomes up to 2 years. *J. Rheumatol.* 37):2362-2368.

[59] Krathen MS, Gottlieb AB, Mease PJ. (2010) Pharmacologic immunomodulation and cutaneous malignancy in rheumatoid arthritis, psoriasis, and psoriatic arthritis. *J. Rheumatol.*37:2205-2215.

[60] McInnes IB, Illei GG, Danning CL, Yarboro CH, Crane M, Kuroiwa T, Schlimgen R, Lee E, Foster B, Flemming D, Prussin C, Fleisher TA, Boumpas DT (2001) IL-10 improves skin disease and modulates endothelial activation and leukocyte effector function in patients with psoriatic arthritis. *J. Immunol.* 167:4075-4082.

[61] Marji JS, Marcus R, Moennich J, Mackay-Wiggan J. (2010) Use of biologic agents in pediatric psoriasis. *J. Drugs Dermatol.* 9:975-86.

[62] Olivieri I, D'Angelo S, Palazzi C, Lubrano E, Leccese P (2010) Emerging drugs for psoriatic arthritis. *Expert Opin. Emerg. Drugs.* 15:399-414.

[63] Saber TP, Ng CT, Renard G, Lynch BM, Pontifex E, Walsh CA, Grier A, Molloy M, Bresnihan B, Fitzgerald O, Fearon U, Veale DJ. (2010)

Remission in psoriatic arthritis: is it possible and how can it be predicted? *Arthritis Res Ther*.12:R94.

[64] Vaz A, Lisse J, Rizzo W, Albani S. (2009) Discussion: DMARDs and biologic therapies in the management of inflammatory joint diseases. *Expert Rev. Clin. Immunol.* 5:291-299.

[65] O'Daly JA, Lezama R, Rodriguez PJ Silva E, Indriago NR, Peña G, Colorado I, Gleason J, Rodríguez B, Acuña L, Ovalles T (2009) Antigens from Leishmania amastigotes induced clinical remission of psoriasis. *Arch. Dermatol. Res.* 301:1-13.

[66] O'Daly JA, Lezama R, Gleason J (2009) Isolation of Leishmania amastigote protein fractions which induced lymphocyte stimulation and remission of psoriasis. *Arch. Dermatol Res.* 301:411-427.

[67] O'Daly JA, Gleason JP, Peña G, Colorado I (2010) Purified proteins from leishmania amastigotes-induced delayed type hypersensitivity reactions and remission of collagen-induced arthritis in animal models. *Arch Dermatol. Res.* 302:567-581.

[68] O'Daly JA, Rodriguez B, Ovalles T, Pelaez C (2010) Lymphocyte subsets in peripheral blood of patients with psoriasis before and after treatment with leishmania antigens. *Arch. Dermatol. Res.* 302:95-104.

[69] O'Daly JA, Gleason J (2010) Antigens from Leishmania amastigotes inducing clinical remission of psoriasis: Relationship between leishmaniasis and psoriasis. *Journal of Clinical Dermatology DERMA* 2010 1:47-57.

[70] O'Daly JA, Gleason J, Lezama R, Rodriguez PJ, Silva E, Indriago NR. Antigens from Leishmania amastigotes inducing clinical remission of psoriatic arthritis. *Archives of Dermatological Research*. In Press February 2011.

In: Arthritis: Types, Treatment and Prevention   ISBN 978-1-61470-719-6
Editor: Marc N. Pelt   © 2012 Nova Science Publishers, Inc.

Chapter III

The Role of Aquaporins in Human Synovitis

Ali Mobasheri[a]*, Christopher A. Moskaluk[b],
David Marples[c] and Mehdi Shakibaei[d]
[a]Division of Veterinary Medicine,
School of Veterinary Medicine and Science,
Faculty of Medicine and Health Sciences,
University of Nottingham, Sutton Bonington Campus, UK
[b]Departments of Pathology, Biochemistry and Molecular Genetics,
University of Virginia Health System, Charlottesville, VA USA
[c]Institute of Membrane and Systems Biology, University of Leeds, UK
[d]Institute of Anatomy, Ludwig-Maximilians-University Munich,
Germany

ABSTRACT

Rheumatoid arthritis (RA) is an autoimmune disorder characterized by synovial proliferation (synovitis), articular cartilage and subchondral bone degradation and synovial inflammation. Joint swelling and oedema

---

* Corresponding author: E-mail: ali.mobasheri@nottingham.ac.uk, Phone: +44-01159516449; Fax; +44-01159516440.

often accompany pannus formation and joint chronic inflammation in RA. Clinical evidence suggests that joint swelling and oedema frequently accompany the chronic inflammation observed in synovial joints of RA patients. Although joint swelling is understood to be a major problem in synovitis, very little is known about the molecular mechanisms responsible for the oedema fluid formation that is associated with joint inflammation. Recent studies from our laboratory have shown that articular chondrocytes and synoviocytes express aquaporin 1 (AQP1) water channels. Aquaporins are a family of small integral membrane proteins related to the major intrinsic protein (MIP or AQP0). In recent studies we have used immunohistochemistry to investigate whether the expression of the AQP1 water channel is altered in synovitis. Our data suggests that this membrane protein is upregulated in the synovium derived from RA and psoriatic arthritis patients. In this chapter these observations are discussed in the context of RA and psoriatic arthritis. AQP1 and other aquaporins may play an important role in joint swelling and the vasogenic oedema fluid formation and hydrarthrosis associated with synovial inflammation.

Keywords: Inflammation; Arthritis; Osteoarthritis; Rheumatoid Arthritis; Synovitis; Aquaporin; Water Channel; Immunohistochemistry

INTRODUCTION

According to the United Nations (UN)[1] and the World Health Organization (WHO)[2] musculoskeletal and arthritic conditions are leading causes of morbidity and disability throughout the world, giving rise to enormous healthcare expenditures and loss of work [1](source: http://www.arthritis.org/)[3] [4]. Many types of rheumatic diseases and arthritic conditions are essentially "inflammatory" disorders. The term "arthritis" characterizes a group of conditions involving inflammatory damage to synovial joints [2]. Arthritis literally means inflammation (*itis*) of the joints (*arthr*). It involves pain, redness, heat, swelling and other harmful effects of inflammation within the joint. There are over 200 different forms of arthritis. The most common form is osteoarthritis (OA) (also known as osteoarthrosis or degenerative joint disease). OA can result from trauma to the joint, infection of

---

[1] www.un.org/
[2] http://www.who.int/en/
[3] http://www.who.int/healthinfo/statistics
[4] http://whqlibdoc.who.int/bulletin/2003/Vol81-No9/bulletin_2003_81(9)_630.pdf

the joint, or simply as a consequence of age. Other forms of arthritis include psoriatic arthritis and rheumatoid arthritis (RA), an autoimmune disease in which the body's own immune system attacks synovial joints.

The UN, the WHO and 37 other countries have proclaimed the year 2000-2010 as the Bone and Joint Decade[5] [1, 3]. This global initiative is intended to improve the lives of people with musculoskeletal disorders, such as arthritis, and to advance understanding and treatment of musculoskeletal disorders through prevention, education and research. The 10-year global initiative launched by the UN urges governments around the world to start taking action to draw attention to the growing pervasiveness and impact of musculoskeletal diseases and to reduce the social and financial burdens to society. Support for this global initiative will raise awareness of musculoskeletal health, stimulate research and improve people's quality of life.

Musculoskeletal diseases are one of the major causes of disability around the world and have been a significant reason for the development of the Bone and Joint Decade [1, 3, 4]. RA, OA, gout and back pain are important causes of loss of disability-adjusted-life years in both the developed and developing world [5].

The Arthritis Foundation[6] in the United States plays a key role in co-ordinating efforts during the Bone and Joint Decade as a supporter. Its aims are to:

– Raise awareness and educate the world on the increasing societal impact of musculoskeletal injuries and disorders
– Empower patients to participate in decisions about their care and treatment
– Increase global funding for prevention activities and treatment research
– Continually seek and promote cost-effective prevention and treatment of musculoskeletal injuries and disorders

The major consequence of all forms of arthritis is joint dysfunction, disability, chronic pain, and significant morbidity. Pain is a constant and daily feature in well-established forms of the disease. Arthritis pain occurs due to inflammation that occurs around the joint, damage to the joint from disease, daily wear and tear of joint, muscular strains caused by movement against

---

[5] http://www.arthritis
[6] http://www.arthritis

stiff, painful joints and fatigue. Disability in patients with arthritis is a consequence of degeneration in the joint and surrounding tissues and is further enhanced by inflammation-induced pain. Aside from analgesics, there are currently no effective pharmacotherapies capable of restoring the structure and function of damaged synovial tissues in any form of arthritis. Consequently, one of the most important factors in treating arthritis is to understand the root causes and find ways to reduce the major risk factors. Many of the root causes of these diseases are presently unknown. Understanding these will allow us to develop better and more targeted therapies with fewer complications and side effects. This chapter will mainly focus on synovial inflammation and oedema and the role of aquaporin water channels in oedema formation and hydrarthrosis. In the following section we will outline the basic structure and function of cartilage and synovium. We will then summarize some of the general features of joint inflammation in OA and RA, before discussing oedema formation and the role of aquaporins in hydrarthrosis.

Anatomy, Histology and Physiology of Articular Cartilage and Synovium

Articular cartilage is a flexible and mechanically compliant connective tissue found at the end of long bones in articulating joints and in the intervertebral disc (Figure 1). Articular cartilage and fibrocartilage differ in the relative amounts of its three principal components, namely collagen fibres, ground substance (proteoglycans) and elastin fibres. Articular cartilage is a load-bearing tissue with unique biological characteristics. Its biochemical properties depend on the structural design of the tissue, the molecular composition of the extracellular matrix (ECM) that makes up the bulk of the tissue volume and the interactions between its resident cells and the ECM [6]. Articular chondrocytes are the only cells found within the cartilage ECM. They are architects of cartilage [7], building the macromolecular framework of its ECM from three distinct classes of macromolecules: collagens (predominantly type II collagens), proteoglycans (mainly aggrecan), and a variety of non-collagenous proteins.

Of the collagens present in articular cartilage collagens type II, IX, and XI form a fibrillar meshwork that gives cartilage tensile stiffness and strength [6, 8, 9], whereas collagen type VI forms part of the matrix immediately surrounding the chondrocytes, enabling them to attach to the macromolecular framework of the ECM and acting as a transducer of biomechanical and biochemical signals in the articular cartilage [10, 11]. Large aggregating proteoglycans (aggrecan) are embedded in the collagen mesh and give cartilage its stiffness to compression, its resilience and contribute to its long-term durability [11-14].

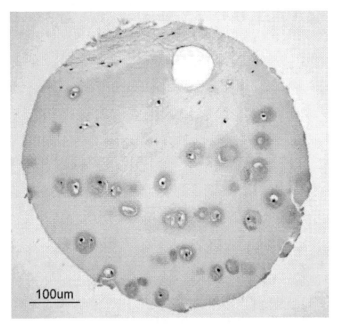

Figure 1. Structure of human articular cartilage. A. This figure illustrates a sample of human cartilage from a tissue microarray developed by the Cooperative Human Tissue Network (CHTN) of the National Cancer Institute (http://www.chtn.nci.nih.gov/). Cartilage is predominantly an avascular, aneural and alymphatic load-bearing connective tissue consisting of a single cell type known as the chondrocyte. Blood vessels are only present in subchondral bone.

ECM proteins in cartilage are of great significance for the regulation of the cell behaviour, proliferation, differentiation and morphogenesis [15-23]. Small proteoglycans, including decorin, biglycan, and fibromodulin are further embedded in the ECM. Decorin and fibromodulin both interact with the type II collagen fibrils in the matrix and have roles in fibrillogenesis and interfibril interactions. Biglycan is mainly found in the area immediately surrounding the chondrocyte, where it may interact with collagen type VI [6, 11]. Modulation of the ECM proteins is regulated by the interaction of a diversity of growth factors with chondrocytes [24-28]. In fact, it has been reported recently, that IGF-I and TGF-β stimulate the chondrocyte surface expression of integrins, and that this event is accompanied by increasing adhesion of chondrocytes to matrix proteins [29]. Other non-collagenous proteins in articular cartilage such as cartilage oligomeric matrix protein (COMP) are less well studied and may have value as biomarkers of cartilage turnover and degeneration of [30], while tenascin and fibronectin influence interactions between the chondrocytes and the ECM [6, 31]. The ECM surrounds chondrocytes; it protects them from the biomechanical stresses that occur during normal joint motion, determines the types and concentrations of molecules that reach the cells and helps to maintain the chondrocyte phenotype.

Throughout life, cartilage is continually remodelled as chondrocytes replace matrix macromolecules lost through degradation. Evidence indicates that ECM turnover depends on the ability of chondrocytes to detect alterations in the macromolecular composition and organization of the matrix, such as the presence of degraded macromolecules, and to respond by synthesizing appropriate types and amounts of new ECM components. It is known that mechanical loading of cartilage creates mechanical, electrical, and physicochemical signals that help to direct the synthesizing and degrading activity of chondrocytes [32]. In addition, the ECM acts as a signal transducer for chondrocytes [33]. A prolonged and severe decrease in the use of the joint leads to alterations in the composition of the ECM and eventually to a loss of tissue structure and its specific biomechanical properties, whereas normal physical strain stimulates the synthesizing activity of chondrocytes and possibly internal tissue remodelling [34, 35].

Although articular cartilage can tolerate a tremendous amount of intensive and repetitive physical stress, it manifests a striking inability to heal even the most minor injury [34, 36-38]. This makes joints particularly sensitive to degenerative processes [39]. Furthermore, aging leads to alterations in ECM composition and alters the activity of the chondrocytes, including their ability to respond to a variety of stimuli such as growth factors [40-42]. All these alterations increase the probability of cartilage degeneration [37, 43-45] and emphasize the importance of interaction of chondrocytes with their surrounding ECM since this interaction regulates their growth, differentiation, and survival [46].

Synovium

The synovium (Figure 2) is a thin layer of specialized connective tissue only a few cells thick. It lines the joints and tendon sheaths and acts to control the environment within the joint and tendon sheath. It does this in two ways: first, it acts as a membrane to determine what can pass into the joint space and what stays outside; second, the cells within the synovium produce synovial fluid and special substances that lubricate and nourish the joint. In the context of this chapter, an important function of the synovium is controlling the volume of fluid in the cavity so that it is just enough to allow the solid components to move over each other freely. This volume is normally so small that the joint is under slight suction.

The synovium inside joints can become irritated, inflamed and thickened in conditions such as such as OA and RA; this is called synovitis. When this happens, the synovium can create additional problems in a variety of ways. Excess synovial fluid weeping from inflamed synovium can provide a barrier to diffusion of nutrients to cartilage.

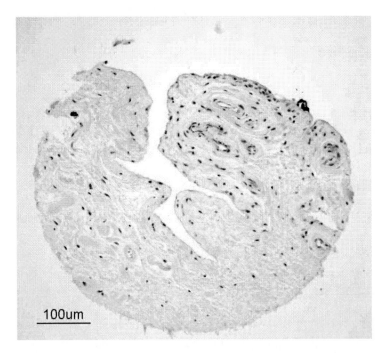

100um

Figure 2. Structure of human synovium. A. This figure illustrates a sample of human synovium from a tissue microarray developed by the Cooperative Human Tissue Network (CHTN) of the National Cancer Institute (http://www.chtn.nci.nih.gov/).

The synovial cells (synoviocytes) may also use up most of the available nutrients so that the glucose levels in the synovial fluid may be significantly diminished. These factors may lead to starvation and eventual apoptotic death of chondrocytes. Synovial cells may also produce enzymes, which can digest the cartilage surface, although it is not clear that these will damage cartilage with healthy cells.

Synovitis can be treated with a variety of medications including non-steroidal anti-inflammatory drugs and corticosterone injections. In some extreme cases the inflamed synovium may be removed using a surgical procedure called synovectomy.

Characteristic Features of OA and RA

This section will summarize some of the general features of OA and RA before moving onto the processes involved in joint inflammation and oedema formation and the role of aquaporins in hydrarthrosis (an effusion of watery liquid into the cavity of a synovial joint).

Osteoarthritis (OA)

OA affects large load-bearing joints and is most problematic in the hip and the knee. The disease is essentially one acquired from daily wear and tear of the joint. Its most prominent feature is the progressive destruction of articular cartilage [47]. OA begins in articular cartilage and eventually spreads to other synovial tissues. The current consensus is that OA is a disease involving not only articular cartilage but also the synovial membrane, subchondral bone and peri-articular soft tissues [48]. OA may occur following traumatic injury to the joint, subsequent to an infection of the joint or simply as a result of aging and the mechanical stresses associated with daily life.

It is now generally accepted that OA must be viewed not only as the final common pathway for aging and injuries of the joint, but also as an active and inflammatory joint disease. As medical advances lengthen average life expectancy, OA will become an even larger public health problem - not only because it is a manifestation of aging but because it usually takes many years to reach clinical relevance. OA is already one of the ten most disabling diseases in industrialized countries. It is one of the most prevalent and chronic diseases affecting the elderly [49]. OA is rare in people under 40 but becomes more common with age – most people over 65 years of age show some radiographic evidence of OA in at least one or more joints. OA is the most frequent cause of physical disability among older adults globally. More than 20 million Americans are estimated to have OA (source: http://www.niams.nih.gov/). It is also anticipated that by the year 2030, 20% of adults will have developed OA in Western Europe and North America.

The symptoms and signs characteristic of OA in the most frequently affected joints are heat, swelling, pain, stiffness and limited mobility. OA is often a progressive and disabling disease, which occurs in the setting of a variety of risk factors, such as advancing age, obesity, and trauma, that conspire to incite a cascade of pathophysiological events within joint tissues [50]. Other important sequelae include osteophyte formation, synovitis and joint swelling [51]. These manifestations are highly variable, depending on joint location and disease severity. Other forms of arthritis include psoriatic arthritis, and autoimmune diseases in which the body's immune system attacks itself such as rheumatoid arthritis (RA). Figure 3 outlines the major molecular and cellular changes that occur in the synovial joint in arthritis and synovitis.

Rheumatoid Arthritis (RA)

In rheumatoid arthritis (RA) the immune system begins an 'autoimmune' attack on synovial joints and other tissues for largely unknown reasons. Most of the damage occurs to the joint lining (synovium) and cartilage, which eventually results in erosion of two opposing bones. RA is a chronic and progressive autoimmune disease [7], [8], [9]. RA affects 0.8-1% of the adult population. It is a painful and chronically disabling condition that can cause severe disability (this varies between individuals and depends on how severe and aggressive the disease is) and ultimately affects a person's ability to carry out even the simplest of everyday tasks.

The disease can progress very rapidly (again the speed of progression varies widely between individuals), causing swelling and damaging cartilage and bone around the joints. Any joint may be affected but it is commonly the hands, feet and wrists.

---

[7]http://www.nras.org.uk/
[8]http://www.nras.org.uk/about_rheumatoid_arthritis
[9]http://www.arthritisresearchuk.org/arthritis

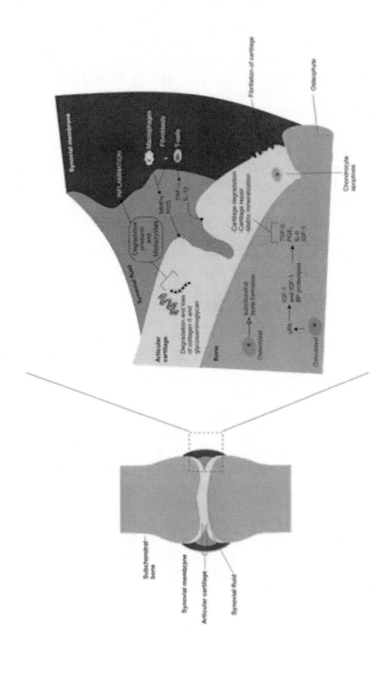

Figure 3. The major molecular and cellular changes that occur in the synovial joint during inflammation.

It is a systemic disease, which means that it can affect the whole body and internal organs such as the lungs, heart and eyes. Furthermore, RA is associated with an increased risk of coronary disease, infection, and lymphoma, as well as reduced life expectancy [52-56]. RA affects approximately 3 times more women than men and onset is generally between 40 - 60 years of age although it can occur at any age.

There are studies that suggest RA is also associated with sex hormone production in the body. The peak incidence of RA in women coincides with the peri-menopausal age, and the juvenile form occurs mainly during puberty, suggesting a connection of RA with hormonal alterations [57]. Although controversial, several studies have reported on ameliorating effects on clinical measures of disease activity and inflammation, improved bone mineral density (BMD), and presented results pointing towards retardation of joint damage by Hormone Replacement Therapy (HRT) [56, 58, 59].

The pathogenesis of RA is very poorly understood and little is known about the risk factors associated with it. Smoking is an important risk factor and makes the outlook much worse but there is no mechanistic insight to explain why this is the case.

There is no cure for RA and more information is needed to help understand about the inflammatory processes that occur in the disease and how to manage it. The effects of RA are not well publicized.

Therefore awareness of the severity of the condition tends to be restricted to those who are directly affected or their carers and relatives. The outlook for RA patients is significantly better now than it was 20-30 years ago.

RA patients will have a much better quality of life especially if the disease is diagnosed and treated with appropriate ant-inflammatory agents. We now know that uncontrolled RA increases mortality through an increased risk of cardiovascular disease such as heart attacks and strokes; again the need for early treatment is imperative. Therefore, we need new and safer drugs for RA and better ways to monitor the disease and avoid prevent noxious stimuli that may cause inflammatory "flare-ups" in the most susceptible individuals.

Effects of Inflammation on Articular Cartilage, Synovium and Other Joint Tissues

As outlined earlier, inflammation is a physiological response that provides protection against an adverse insult or injury and is used to remove the agents causing the inflammation and promote the repair of damaged tissues. When the causative agent cannot be destroyed, for instance, in a RA joint, chronic inflammation results in extensive damage to joint tissues. Additionally tissue- and cell-derived factors in an inflammatory response contribute to the destruction of joint tissues. These include lysosomal enzymes released by inflammatory cells and macrophages [60, 61], reactive oxygen species [62, 63], prostaglandins and pro-inflammatory cytokines [64]. These factors have been suggested to play a central role in the degeneration of articular cartilage during inflammation of the joint [65]. The main symptom of joint inflammation in OA is pain, which is actually a physiological signal to the brain and the immune system to protect the joint from extreme use.

Joint damage causes inflammation and stimulates the synthesis and release of more mediators that degrade joint tissues [66]. Several studies have reported that pro-inflammatory cytokines induce hyperplasia of synovial cells (i.e. synovitis) in joints. This is an important aetiology for RA; high concentrations of TNF-α and IL-1β have been reported within the synovial fluid and plasma of patients with RA [67, 68].

Pro-inflammatory cytokines stimulate the synthesis of matrix metalloproteinases, activate caspase-3 (and downstream effector caspases) and stimulate osteoclasts, causing irreversible damage to soft and calcified tissues (i.e. subchondral bone) in joints [69, 70]. Furthermore, cytokines suppress the expression of cartilage-specific ECM components in chondrocytes such as collagen type II and cartilage-specific proteoglycans exacerbating the arthritis associated loss of cartilage ECM [71-73].

Chondrocyte proliferation is considered to be an attempt to counteract cartilage degradation but disease progression and secondary inflammation proves that this is generally unsuccessful. The short-lived hyperplasia (chondrocyte cloning) is followed by hypocellularity and apoptosis [74-78]. Catabolic events responsible for cartilage matrix degradation comprise the release of catabolic cytokines such as IL-1β, IL-6 and TNF-α [79, 80] inducing matrix degrading enzymes such as matrix metalloproteinases (MMPs) and aggrecanase (ADAM-TS4, ADAM-TS11) by chondrocytes and by synoviocytes in early OA [79-83]. An imbalance between MMPs and tissue inhibitors of MMPs occurs, resulting in active MMPs and this may be important in cartilage matrix degradation. However, IL-1β may also contribute to the depletion of cartilage matrix by decreasing synthesis of cartilage specific proteoglycans and collagen type II [73, 82, 84, 85]. Systemic effects of elevated IL-1β levels include stimulation of glucose transport and metabolism causing hypoglycaemia and impairing glucose-induced insulin secretion (86). In articular cartilage, the acute effects of IL-1β also involve stimulated glucose uptake and metabolism [87, 88]. When the matrix is degraded, an inappropriate, inferior repair matrix is synthesized which cannot withstand mechanical load. Consequently, cartilage fibrillation and breakdown occurs by the focal formation of vertical, oblique and tangential clefts into the ECM and is localized preferentially in areas of proteoglycan depletion. Apoptosis is another contributing factor to the loss of articular cartilage in RA and OA: apoptosis increases the cell loss observed in aging and OA cartilage [74, 78, 89].

Many of the biological effects of pro-inflammatory cytokines on chondrocytes have been shown to be regulated by the ubiquitous central transcription factor NF-κB [90-92]. In other cell types the expression of adhesion molecules such as cell adhesion molecule-I (I-CAM), vascular endothelial growth factor (VEGF), urokinase plasmin activator (uPa), Bcl-2 and pro-inflammatory cytokines have been shown to be regulated by NF-κB [93-95]. NF-κB appears to be a common downstream target of multiple converging catabolic signaling pathways (e.g. those mediated by IL-1β and TNF-α (96). NF-κB is present in the cytoplasm as an inactive heterotrimer complex consisting of two subunits and an additional inhibitory subunit: IκBα. Five different subunits exist: c-Rel, RelA (also known as p65), RelB, p50/p105, p52/p100, which can form homo or heterodimers in varying combinations. P65/p50 is one of the most prevalent combinations [97]. During the activation process, the inhibitory subunit IκBα is phosphorylated at Ser 32 and Ser 36 residues by IKK kinase (IκBα kinase) and is subsequently degraded. Once released, subunits of activated NF-κB translocate to the nucleus where they bind NF-κB-recognition (κB) sites in the promoter regions of selected target genes, activating their expression [90, 98]. Dysregulation of NF-κB has been implicated in the pathogenesis of a wide spectrum of human diseases including cancer, Alzheimer's disease, multiple sclerosis, cardiovascular disease and RA [97]. Activation of NF-κB has been observed in synovial cells from patients with RA [99].

Aquaporin Water Channels

Aquaporins are a family of membrane bound proteins that are extensively distributed in microorganisms (100), animals [101-103] and plants [104-106]. They are small integral membrane proteins that are expressed in a variety of epithelial tissues where they are responsible for regulating rapid water movement across epithelial barriers driven by osmotic gradients. Aquaporins play fundamental roles in water and small solute transport across epithelial and endothelial barriers [107, 108]

In mammals, aquaporins are located at strategic membrane sites in endothelia and a variety of epithelia, most of which have well-defined physiological functions in fluid absorption or secretion [109]. To date, 13 members of the aquaporin gene family have been identified in humans: AQP0-AQP12 (110). Animal genome projects have also confirmed the presence of multiple aquaporin genes encoding distinct protein isoforms. The proteins encoded by aquaporin genes have been classified into two major groups based on their substrate permeabilities:

1) the classical water permeable aquaporins are permeated by water and include AQP1, AQP2, AQP4, AQP5 and AQP8 [101];
2) the water and small solute permeable aquaglyceroporins exhibit permeability to water and a range of small neutral solutes.

These may include substances such as glycerol and urea. Aquaglyceroporins include AQP3, AQP7, AQP9 and AQP10 [101, 111].

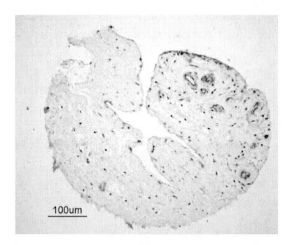

Figure 4. Expression of AQP1 in the human synovium. The tissue section shown in this figure is from a tissue microarray developed by the Cooperative Human Tissue Network (CHTN) of the National Cancer Institute (http://www.chtn.nci.nih.gov/). The section was immunostained using affinity purified polyclonal antibodies to rat AQP1. The polyclonal antibody used has been shown to exhibit broad mammalian cross-reactivity.

Immunolocalization of Aquaporin 1 in Human Cartilage and Synovium

Until recently nothing was known about the expression of aquaporins in cartilage and synovium. Recent immunohistochemical studies from our laboratories have confirmed the presence of aquaporins in human and equine articular cartilage [112, 113] and human synovial tissues [114].

Our work in human intervertebral disc has provided evidence for the presence of AQP1 and AQP3 [115]. Using human tissue microarray in immunohistochemical studies has allowed us to confirm the expression of AQP1 [114] and AQP3 [116] in human synovium (see Figures 4 and 5).

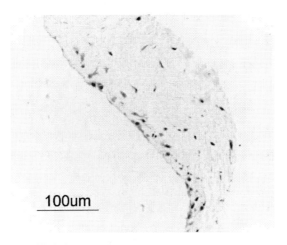

100um

Figure 5. Expression of AQP3 in the human synovium. The tissue section shown in this figure is from a tissue microarray developed by the Cooperative Human Tissue Network (CHTN) of the National Cancer Institute (http://www.chtn.nci.nih.gov/). It was immunostained using a commercially produced affinity purified polyclonal antibody to rat AQP3.

Physiological Relevance of Synovial Aquaporins to Synovial Oedema

Rheumatoid arthritis (RA) is a systemic and often chronically progressive inflammatory disorder of unknown aetiology that affects many tissues and organs in approximately 1% of the human population. RA principally attacks the joints producing a symmetric polyarthritis associated with swelling and pain in multiple joints [117]. The inflammatory synovitis that accompanies RA often progresses to destruction of the articular cartilage and ankylosis of the joints. Thus RA may exhibit a painful, chronic, and fluctuating course, resulting in permanent disability, significant morbidity and increased mortality. Active inflammation is a key feature of RA and is first seen in the synovial membranes of the joints, which become red and swollen. The earliest structural abnormalities in RA consist of proliferation of the synovial lining ('synovitis'), soft tissue swelling [118], and osteoporosis. In later stages, a layer of roughened and inflamed synovial granulation tissue, known as the pannus, protrudes over the surface of the articular cartilage. Under the pannus the cartilage is actively eroded, leading to massive chondral and small bone erosions. The joints become fixed in place (ankylosed) by the thickened and hardened pannus, which also may cause displacement and deformity of the joint. The formation and maintenance of the invasive pannus in RA is an integral part of disease progression since it exacerbates articular inflammation causing cartilage degradation, bone erosion and joint swelling [119].

Recent studies suggest that the synovial vasculature and endothelial mitogens such as vascular endothelial growth factor (VEGF) play an important role in this process [120]. In the normal joint the synovial micro-vasculature delivers essential nutrients and oxygen to the synovial tissues. In synovitis the same synovial micro-vasculature is thought to be responsible for delivery of pro-inflammatory cytokines (i.e. TNFα and IL-1β) and inflammatory cells (polymorphonuclear and mononuclear leukocytes) to the inflamed and swollen synovium. A vicious cycle of altered cytokine and signal transduction pathways then ensues, which results in inhibition of apoptotic programmed cell death in synoviocytes and contributes to synoviocyte and osteoclast mediated cartilage and bone destruction. Selective inhibition of pro-inflammatory cytokines [121] and blockade of VEGF activity [120, 122] and angiogenesis [123] have been suggested to attenuate RA in animal studies. These observations indicate that pro-inflammatory cytokines, angiogenic factors and synovial micro-vessels are integral to the development of synovitis and the sustained progression of RA.

Although joint swelling is understood to be a major problem in synovitis, virtually nothing is known about the molecular mechanisms responsible for the oedema fluid formation that is associated with joint inflammation. Recent studies from our laboratories have shown that articular chondrocytes and synoviocytes express aquaporin 1 (AQP1) water channels [112, 113, 124]. The aquaporins are a family of small integral membrane proteins related to the major intrinsic protein (MIP or AQP0) [125, 126]. AQP1 is a relatively well-characterized membrane protein, which belongs to the aquaporin family of proteins and is selectively permeated by water driven by osmotic gradients [101]. AQP1 is abundantly expressed in human erythrocytes, micro-vascular endothelia and renal proximal tubules (apical and basolateral membrane domain of proximal tubule cells), thin descending limbs of the loop of Henle [127]. AQP1 is expressed in many epithelial and endothelial barriers as well as other tissues [108, 128, 129]. AQP1 is also present in many other tissues including choroid plexus (apical membranes of epithelial cells), gallbladder, pancreatic ducts, intrahepatic cholangiocytes, hepatic ducts, placenta, amniotic membranes, cartilage and synovium [112].

We presented the first molecular and immunohistochemical evidence for the presence of AQP1 in cartilage and synovium in 2004 [112, 113, 124] and showed that AQP1 is upregulated in articular cartilage from RA patients [124]. We speculated whether its expression may be altered in the synovium in inflammatory synovitis and hydrarthrosis. Joint swelling and hydrarthrosis accompany the chronic inflammation seen in RA, which results in the oedematous formation of a watery effusion in the joint cavity. To test this hypothesis, we used immunohistochemistry to compare the expression of AQP1 water channels in normal human synovium with human synovitis samples on commercially available synovitis Tissue MicroArrays (TMAs) to determine if AQP1 expression is altered in the synovitis and whether the hydrarthrosis associated with RA could be a result of increased AQP1 expression in the synovium [114]. Immunohistochemistry revealed that AQP1 is expressed in synovial micro-vessels and synoviocytes from normal joints. Semi-quantitative histomorphometric analysis of AQP1 expression in the TMAs revealed upregulation of the membrane protein in the synovium derived from RA and psoriatic arthritis patients [114]. These results indicate a potential role for synovial AQP1 and other aquaporins in joint swelling and the vasogenic oedema fluid formation and hydrarthrosis associated with synovial inflammation. These results also support the idea that the oedema formation and synovial fluid accumulation in RA joints may be a consequence of elevated AQP1 expression in the synovium, a new observation that has not been made previously.

CONCLUSIONS

In oedema, either too much fluid moves from the blood vessels into the tissues, or not enough fluid moves from the tissues back into the blood vessels. This fluid imbalance can cause mild to severe swelling in one or more parts of the body. We have recently shown that AQP1 is expressed in normal human chondrocytes and synoviocytes [112]. In parallel studies we demonstrated that AQP1 expression is increased in chondrocytes and synoviocytes from RA cartilage [114, 124]. Our data suggests a potential role for AQP1 in the formation of vasogenic oedema fluid formation and joint swelling associated with synovial inflammation in RA.

We have also studied the expression of two aquaglyceroporins (AQP3 and AQP9) in normal and synovitis synovium (Mobasheri et al., unpublished observations). Preliminary immunohistochemical studies suggest that the expression of these two aquaglyceroporins is also increased in human synovitis. However, whether they are also involved in joint swelling and hydrarthrosis in synovitis remains to be determined. Future studies will also need to employ more quantitative methods for studying the expression of aquaporins and aquaglyceroporins in RA samples. This can be done using the same semi-quantitative approach that we have recently adopted for studying the expression of AQP1 in RA joints [124]. Regulation of aquaporin expression by pro-inflammatory cytokines in cultured synovial cells *in vitro* will also be the subject of functional experiments in future investigations.

The studies reviewed in this chapter highlight the importance of oedema formation in synovial inflammation and suggest that several aquaporin proteins are involved in synovial oedema formation. Future studies will need to determine if additional aquaporins are involved at different stages of joint inflammation and correlate the expression of these with the formation of synovial oedema. A better understanding of the molecular mechanisms involved in synovial fluid accumulation may allow us to develop new anti-inflammatory therapies to prevent or significantly reduce oedema. Further work is required to develop a larger bank of synovial tissue samples for more comprehensive immunohistochemical analysis using custom designed tissue micro-arrays. It will also be useful to obtain further information about aquaporin expression in other types of inflammatory arthritis.

ACKNOWLEDGMENTS

Dr. A. Mobasheri acknowledges the financial support of The Wellcome Trust, the National Centre for the Replacement, Refinement and Reduction of Animals in Research (NC3Rs) (grant number: Mobasheri.A.28102007), the Biotechnology and Biological Sciences Research Council (BBSRC) (grants BBSRC/S/M/2006/ 13141 and BB/G018030/1), the Engineering and Physical Sciences Research Council (EPSRC). We would like to thank all members of our laboratories for their support and collaboration. We thank Dr. Madura "Dexter" Batuwangala for providing the illustration in Figure 3.

REFERENCES

[1]   Woolf AD, Pfleger B. Burden of major musculoskeletal conditions. *Bull World Health Organ.* 2003;81(9):646-56.

[2]   Di Paola R, Cuzzocrea S. Predictivity and sensitivity of animal models of arthritis. *Autoimmun. Rev.* 2008 Oct;8(1):73-5.

[3]   McGowan JA. Perspectives on the future of bone and joint diseases. *J. Rheumatol. Suppl.* 2003 Aug;67:62-4.

[4]   Brooks PM. Impact of osteoarthritis on individuals and society: how much disability? Social consequences and health economic implications. *Curr. Opin. Rheumatol.* 2002 Sep;14(5):573-7.

[5]   Brooks PM. The burden of musculoskeletal disease--a global perspective. *Clin. Rheumatol.* 2006 Nov;25(6):778-81.

[6]   Buckwalter JA, Mankin HJ. Articular cartilage: tissue design and chondrocyte-matrix interactions. *Instr Course Lect.* 1998;47:477-86.

[7]   Muir H. The chondrocyte, architect of cartilage. Biomechanics, structure, function and molecular biology of cartilage matrix macromolecules. *Bioessays.* 1995 Dec;17(12):1039-48.

[8]   Eyre DR. Collagens and cartilage matrix homeostasis. *Clin. Orthop. Relat. Res.* 2004 Oct(427 Suppl):S118-22.

[9]   Kuettner KE, Aydelotte MB, Thonar EJ. Articular cartilage matrix and structure: a minireview. *J. Rheumatol. Suppl.* 1991 Feb;27:46-8.

[10] Guilak F, Alexopoulos LG, Upton ML, Youn I, Choi JB, Cao L, et al. The pericellular matrix as a transducer of biomechanical and biochemical signals in articular cartilage. *Ann. N Y Acad. Sci.* 2006 Apr;1068:498-512.

[11] Roughley PJ, Lee ER. Cartilage proteoglycans: structure and potential functions. *Microsc. Res. Tech.* 1994 Aug 1;28(5):385-97.

[12] Dudhia J. Aggrecan, aging and assembly in articular cartilage. *Cell Mol. Life Sci.* 2005 Oct;62(19-20):2241-56.

[13] Kiani C, Chen L, Wu YJ, Yee AJ, Yang BB. Structure and function of aggrecan. *Cell Res.* 2002 Mar;12(1):19-32.

[14] Luo W, Guo C, Zheng J, Chen TL, Wang PY, Vertel BM, et al. Aggrecan from start to finish. *J. Bone Miner Metab.* 2000;18(2):51-6.

[15] Kosher RA, Lash JW, Minor RR. Environmental enhancement of in vitro chondrogenesis. IV. Stimulation of somite chondrogenesis by exogenous chondromucoprotein. *Developmental biology.* 1973 Dec;35(2):210-20.

[16] Kosher RA, Church RL. Stimulation of in vitro somite chondrogenesis by procollagen and collagen. *Nature.* 1975 Nov 27;258(5533):327-30.

[17] von der Mark K, Gauss V, von der Mark H, Muller P. Relationship between cell shape and type of collagen synthesised as chondrocytes lose their cartilage phenotype in culture. *Nature.* 1977 Jun 9;267(5611):531-2.

[18] Hewitt AT, Varner HH, Silver MH, Martin GR. The role of chondronectin and cartilage proteoglycan in the attachment of chondrocytes to collagen. *Progress in clinical and biological research.* 1982;110 Pt B:25-33.

[19] Sommarin Y, Larsson T, Heinegard D. Chondrocyte-matrix interactions. Attachment to proteins isolated from cartilage. *Experimental cell research.* 1989 Sep;184(1):181-92.

[20] Ramachandrula A, Tiku K, Tiku ML. Tripeptide RGD-dependent adhesion of articular chondrocytes to synovial fibroblasts. *Journal of cell science.* 1992 Apr;101 (Pt 4):859-71.

[21] Ruoslahti E, Reed JC. Anchorage dependence, integrins, and apoptosis. *Cell.* 1994 May 20;77(4):477-8.

[22] Enomoto-Iwamoto M, Iwamoto M, Nakashima K, Mukudai Y, Boettiger D, Pacifici M, et al. Involvement of alpha5beta1 integrin in matrix interactions and proliferation of chondrocytes. *J. Bone Miner Res.* 1997 Jul;12(7):1124-32.

[23] Gonzalez FA, Seth A, Raden DL, Bowman DS, Fay FS, Davis RJ. Serum-induced translocation of mitogen-activated protein kinase to the cell surface ruffling membrane and the nucleus. *The Journal of cell biology*. 1993 Sep;122(5):1089-101.

[24] Jenniskens YM, Koevoet W, de Bart AC, Weinans H, Jahr H, Verhaar JA, et al. Biochemical and functional modulation of the cartilage collagen network by IGF1, TGFbeta2 and FGF2. Osteoarthritis and cartilage / OARS, Osteoarthritis Research Society. 2006 Nov; 14(11): 1136-46.

[25] Trippel SB, Corvol MT, Dumontier MF, Rappaport R, Hung HH, Mankin HJ. Effect of somatomedin-C/insulin-like growth factor I and growth hormone on cultured growth plate and articular chondrocytes. *Pediatric research*. 1989 Jan;25(1):76-82.

[26] Isgaard J. Expression and regulation of IGF-I in cartilage and skeletal muscle. *Growth regulation*. 1992 Mar;2(1):16-22.

[27] Hunziker EB, Wagner J, Zapf J. Differential effects of insulin-like growth factor I and growth hormone on developmental stages of rat growth plate chondrocytes in vivo. *The Journal of clinical investigation*. 1994 Mar;93(3):1078-86.

[28] Sah RL, Chen AC, Grodzinsky AJ, Trippel SB. Differential effects of bFGF and IGF-I on matrix metabolism in calf and adult bovine cartilage explants. *Archives of biochemistry and biophysics*. 1994 Jan;308(1):137-47.

[29] Loeser RF. Growth factor regulation of chondrocyte integrins. Differential effects of insulin-like growth factor 1 and transforming growth factor beta on alpha 1 beta 1 integrin expression and chondrocyte adhesion to type VI collagen. *Arthritis and rheumatism*. 1997 Feb;40(2):270-6.

[30] Di Cesare PE, Carlson CS, Stolerman ES, Hauser N, Tulli H, Paulsson M. Increased degradation and altered tissue distribution of cartilage oligomeric matrix protein in human rheumatoid and osteoarthritic cartilage. *J. Orthop. Res.* 1996 Nov;14(6):946-55.

[31] Burton-Wurster N, Lust G, Macleod JN. Cartilage fibronectin isoforms: in search of functions for a special population of matrix glycoproteins. *Matrix Biol.* 1997 Mar;15(7):441-54.

[32] Mobasheri A, Carter SD, Martin-Vasallo P, Shakibaei M. Integrins and stretch activated ion channels; putative components of functional cell surface mechanoreceptors in articular chondrocytes. *Cell Biol. Int.* 2002;26(1):1-18.

[33] Millward-Sadler SJ, Salter DM. Integrin-dependent signal cascades in chondrocyte mechanotransduction. *Ann. Biomed. Eng.* 2004 Mar;32(3):435-46.

[34] Buckwalter JA, Lane NE. Athletics and osteoarthritis. Am J Sports Med. 1997 Nov-Dec;25(6):873-81.

[35] Maffulli N, King JB. Effects of physical activity on some components of the skeletal system. *Sports Med.* 1992 Jun;13(6):393-407.

[36] Martin JA, Brown T, Heiner A, Buckwalter JA. Post-traumatic osteoarthritis: the role of accelerated chondrocyte senescence. *Biorheology.* 2004;41(3-4):479-91.

[37] Buckwalter JA. Sports, joint injury, and posttraumatic osteoarthritis. *J. Orthop. Sports Phys. Ther.* 2003 Oct;33(10):578-88.

[38] Newman AP. Articular cartilage repair. *Am. J. Sports Med.* 1998 Mar-Apr;26(2):309-24.

[39] Solursh M. Formation of cartilage tissue in vitro. *J. Cell Biochem.* 1991 Mar;45(3):258-60.

[40] Hudelmaier M, Glaser C, Hohe J, Englmeier KH, Reiser M, Putz R, et al. Age-related changes in the morphology and deformational behavior of knee joint cartilage. *Arthritis and rheumatism.* 2001 Nov;44(11):2556-61.

[41] Eckstein F, Reiser M, Englmeier KH, Putz R. In vivo morphometry and functional analysis of human articular cartilage with quantitative magnetic resonance imaging--from image to data, from data to theory. *Anat Embryol.* (Berl). 2001 Mar;203(3):147-73.

[42] Ralphs JR, Benjamin M. The joint capsule: structure, composition, ageing and disease. *J. Anat.* 1994 Jun;184 (Pt 3):503-9.

[43] Sarzi-Puttini P, Cimmino MA, Scarpa R, Caporali R, Parazzini F, Zaninelli A, et al. Osteoarthritis: an overview of the disease and its treatment strategies. *Semin Arthritis Rheum.* 2005 Aug;35(1 Suppl 1):1-10.

[44] Poole AR. An introduction to the pathophysiology of osteoarthritis. *Front Biosci.* 1999 Oct 15;4:D662-70.

[45] Setton LA, Elliott DM, Mow VC. Altered mechanics of cartilage with osteoarthritis: human osteoarthritis and an experimental model of joint degeneration. *Osteoarthritis Cartilage.* 1999 Jan;7(1):2-14.

[46] Shakibaei M, John T, De Souza P, Rahmanzadeh R, Merker HJ. Signal transduction by beta1 integrin receptors in human chondrocytes in vitro: collaboration with the insulin-like growth factor-I receptor. *Biochem. J.* 1999 Sep 15;342 Pt 3:615-23.

[47] Buckwalter JA, Mankin HJ, Grodzinsky AJ. Articular cartilage and osteoarthritis. *Instr. Course Lect.* 2005;54:465-80.

[48] Goldring MB, Goldring SR. Osteoarthritis. *J. Cell Physiol.* 2007 Dec;213(3):626-34.

[49] Aigner T, Rose J, Martin J, Buckwalter J. Aging theories of primary osteoarthritis: from epidemiology to molecular biology. *Rejuvenation Res.* 2004 Summer;7(2):134-45.

[50] Abramson SB, Attur M. Developments in the scientific understanding of osteoarthritis. *Arthritis Res. Ther.* 2009;11(3):227.

[51] Sutton S, Clutterbuck A, Harris P, Gent T, Freeman S, Foster N, et al. The contribution of the synovium, synovial derived inflammatory cytokines and neuropeptides to the pathogenesis of osteoarthritis. *Vet. J.* 2009 Jan;179(1):10-24.

[52] Wolfe F, Michaud K. The effect of methotrexate and anti-tumor necrosis factor therapy on the risk of lymphoma in rheumatoid arthritis in 19,562 patients during 89,710 person-years of observation. *Arthritis Rheum.* 2007 May;56(5):1433-9.

[53] Wolfe F, Michaud K. Lymphoma in rheumatoid arthritis: the effect of methotrexate and anti-tumor necrosis factor therapy in 18,572 patients. *Arthritis Rheum.* 2004 Jun;50(6):1740-51.

[54] Pinals RS. Survival in rheumatoid arthritis. *Arthritis Rheum.* 1987 Apr;30(4):473-5.

[55] Reilly PA, Cosh JA, Maddison PJ, Rasker JJ, Silman AJ. Mortality and survival in rheumatoid arthritis: a 25 year prospective study of 100 patients. *Ann. Rheum. Dis.* 1990 Jun;49(6):363-9.

[56] Mitchell DM, Spitz PW, Young DY, Bloch DA, McShane DJ, Fries JF. Survival, prognosis, and causes of death in rheumatoid arthritis. *Arthritis Rheum.* 1986 Jun;29(6):706-14.

[57] Goemaere S, Ackerman C, Goethals K, De Keyser F, Van der Straeten C, Verbruggen G, et al. Onset of symptoms of rheumatoid arthritis in relation to age, sex and menopausal transition. *J. Rheumatol.* 1990 Dec;17(12):1620-2.

[58] D'Elia HF, Larsen A, Mattsson LA, Waltbrand E, Kvist G, Mellstrom D, et al. Influence of hormone replacement therapy on disease progression and bone mineral density in rheumatoid arthritis. *J. Rheumatol.* 2003 Jul;30(7):1456-63.

[59] D'Elia HF, Mattsson LA, Ohlsson C, Nordborg E, Carlsten H. Hormone replacement therapy in rheumatoid arthritis is associated with lower

serum levels of soluble IL-6 receptor and higher insulin-like growth factor 1. *Arthritis Res Ther.* 2003;5(4):R202-9.

[60] Bartholomew JS, Lowther DA, Handley CJ. Changes in proteoglycan biosynthesis following leukocyte elastase treatment of bovine articular cartilage in culture. *Arthritis Rheum.* 1984 Aug;27(8):905-12.

[61] Cooke TD, Sumi M, Maeda M. Nicolas Andry Award, 1984. Deleterious interactions of immune complexes in cartilage of experimental immune arthritis. I. The erosion of pannus-free hyaline cartilage. *Clin. Orthop Relat Res.* 1985 Mar(193):235-45.

[62] Schalkwijk J, van den Berg WB, van de Putte LB, Joosten LA. An experimental model for hydrogen peroxide-induced tissue damage. Effects of a single inflammatory mediator on (peri)articular tissues. *Arthritis Rheum.* 1986 Apr;29(4):532-8.

[63] Schalkwijk J, van den Berg WB, van de Putte LB, Joosten LA. An experimental model for hydrogen peroxide induced tissue damage: effect on cartilage and other articular tissues. *Int. J. Tissue React.* 1987;9(1):39-43.

[64] Pettipher ER, Higgs GA, Henderson B. Interleukin 1 induces leukocyte infiltration and cartilage proteoglycan degradation in the synovial joint. *Proc. Natl. Acad. Sci. USA.* 1986 Nov;83(22):8749-53.

[65] Keiser H, Greenwald RA, Feinstein G, Janoff A. Degradation of cartilage proteoglycan by human leukocyte granule neutral proteases--a model of joint injury. II. Degradation of isolated bovine nasal cartilage proteoglycan. *J. Clin. Invest.* 1976 Mar;57(3):625-32.

[66] Calin A. Clinical aspects of the effect of NSAID on cartilage. *J. Rheumatol. Suppl.* 1989 Aug;18:43-4.

[67] Eastgate JA, Symons JA, Wood NC, Grinlinton FM, di Giovine FS, Duff GW. Correlation of plasma interleukin 1 levels with disease activity in rheumatoid arthritis. *Lancet.* 1988 Sep 24;2(8613):706-9.

[68] Saxne T, Palladino MA, Jr., Heinegard D, Talal N, Wollheim FA. Detection of tumor necrosis factor alpha but not tumor necrosis factor beta in rheumatoid arthritis synovial fluid and serum. *Arthritis Rheum.* 1988 Aug;31(8):1041-5.

[69] Csaki C, Mobasheri A, Shakibaei M. Synergistic chondroprotective effects of curcumin and resveratrol in human articular chondrocytes: inhibition of IL-1beta-induced NF-kappaB-mediated inflammation and apoptosis. *Arthritis Res Ther.* 2009;11(6):R165.

[70] Olsen NJ, Stein CM. New drugs for rheumatoid arthritis. *N. Engl. J. Med.* 2004 May 20;350(21):2167-79.

[71] Kolettas E, Muir HI, Barrett JC, Hardingham TE. Chondrocyte phenotype and cell survival are regulated by culture conditions and by specific cytokines through the expression of Sox-9 transcription factor. *Rheumatology* (Oxford). 2001 Oct;40(10):1146-56.

[72] Murakami S, Lefebvre V, de Crombrugghe B. Potent inhibition of the master chondrogenic factor Sox9 gene by interleukin-1 and tumor necrosis factor-alpha. *J. Biol. Chem.* 2000 Feb 4;275(5):3687-92.

[73] Robbins JR, Thomas B, Tan L, Choy B, Arbiser JL, Berenbaum F, et al. Immortalized human adult articular chondrocytes maintain cartilage-specific phenotype and responses to interleukin-1beta. *Arthritis Rheum.* 2000 Oct;43(10):2189-201.

[74] Blanco FJ, Guitian R, Vazquez-Martul E, de Toro FJ, Galdo F. Osteoarthritis chondrocytes die by apoptosis. A possible pathway for osteoarthritis pathology. *Arthritis Rheum.* 1998 Feb;41(2):284-9.

[75] Blanco FJ, Ochs RL, Schwarz H, Lotz M. Chondrocyte apoptosis induced by nitric oxide. *Am. J. Pathol.* 1995 Jan;146(1):75-85.

[76] Clegg PD, Mobasheri A. Chondrocyte apoptosis, inflammatory mediators and equine osteoarthritis. *Vet. J.* 2003 Jul;166(1):3-4.

[77] Kim DY, Taylor HW, Moore RM, Paulsen DB, Cho DY. Articular chondrocyte apoptosis in equine osteoarthritis. *Vet. J.* 2003 Jul;166(1):52-7.

[78] Mobasheri A. Role of chondrocyte death and hypocellularity in ageing human articular cartilage and the pathogenesis of osteoarthritis. *Med. Hypotheses.* 2002 Mar;58(3):193-7.

[79] Goldring MB. The role of cytokines as inflammatory mediators in osteoarthritis: lessons from animal models. *Connect Tissue Res.* 1999;40(1):1-11.

[80] Westacott CI, Sharif M. Cytokines in osteoarthritis: mediators or markers of joint destruction? *Semin. Arthritis Rheum.* 1996 Feb;25(4):254-72.

[81] Goldring MB. The role of the chondrocyte in osteoarthritis. *Arthritis Rheum.* 2000 Sep;43(9):1916-26.

[82] Goldring MB. Osteoarthritis and cartilage: the role of cytokines. *Curr. Rheumatol. Rep.* 2000 Dec;2(6):459-65.

[83] Martel-Pelletier J. Pathophysiology of osteoarthritis. *Osteoarthritis Cartilage.* 1998 Nov;6(6):374-6.

[84] Richardson DW, Dodge GR. Effects of interleukin-1beta and tumor necrosis factor-alpha on expression of matrix-related genes by cultured equine articular chondrocytes. *Am. J. Vet. Res.* 2000 Jun;61(6):624-30.

[85] Studer RK, Georgescu HI, Miller LA, Evans CH. Inhibition of transforming growth factor beta production by nitric oxide-treated chondrocytes: implications for matrix synthesis. *Arthritis Rheum.* 1999 Feb;42(2):248-57.

[86] del Rey A, Besedovsky H. Interleukin 1 affects glucose homeostasis. *Am. J. Physiol.* 1987 Nov;253(5 Pt 2):R794-8.

[87] Hernvann A, Jaffray P, Hilliquin P, Cazalet C, Menkes CJ, Ekindjian OG. Interleukin-1 beta-mediated glucose uptake by chondrocytes. Inhibition by cortisol. *Osteoarthritis Cartilage.* 1996 Jun;4(2):139-42.

[88] Shikhman AR, Brinson DC, Valbracht J, Lotz MK. Cytokine regulation of facilitated glucose transport in human articular chondrocytes. *J. Immunol.* 2001 Dec 15;167(12):7001-8.

[89] Adams CS, Horton WE, Jr. Chondrocyte apoptosis increases with age in the articular cartilage of adult animals. *Anat. Rec.* 1998 Apr;250(4):418-25.

[90] Largo R, Alvarez-Soria MA, Diez-Ortego I, Calvo E, Sanchez-Pernaute O, Egido J, et al. Glucosamine inhibits IL-1beta-induced NFkappaB activation in human osteoarthritic chondrocytes. *Osteoarthritis Cartilage.* 2003 Apr;11(4):290-8.

[91] Liacini A, Sylvester J, Li WQ, Huang W, Dehnade F, Ahmad M, et al. Induction of matrix metalloproteinase-13 gene expression by TNF-alpha is mediated by MAP kinases, AP-1, and NF-kappaB transcription factors in articular chondrocytes. *Exp. Cell Res.* 2003 Aug 1;288(1):208-17.

[92] Singh S. From exotic spice to modern drug? *Cell.* 2007 Sep 7;130(5):765-8.

[93] Bharti AC, Aggarwal BB. Nuclear factor-kappa B and cancer: its role in prevention and therapy. *Biochem. Pharmacol.* 2002 Sep;64(5-6):883-8.

[94] Crawford MJ, Krishnamoorthy RR, Rudick VL, Collier RJ, Kapin M, Aggarwal BB, et al. Bcl-2 overexpression protects photooxidative stress-induced apoptosis of photoreceptor cells via NF-kappaB preservation. *Biochem. Biophys. Res. Commun.* 2001 Mar;281(5):1304-12.

[95] Shakibaei M, Csaki C, Nebrich S, Mobasheri A. Resveratrol suppresses interleukin-1beta-induced inflammatory signaling and apoptosis in human articular chondrocytes: potential for use as a novel nutraceutical for the treatment of osteoarthritis. *Biochem. Pharmacol.* 2008 Dec 1;76(11):1426-39.

[96] Feldmann M, Andreakos E, Smith C, Bondeson J, Yoshimura S, Kiriakidis S, et al. Is NF-kappaB a useful therapeutic target in rheumatoid arthritis? *Ann. Rheum. Dis.* 2002 Nov;61 Suppl 2:ii13-8.

[97] Kumar A, Takada Y, Boriek AM, Aggarwal BB. Nuclear factor-kappaB: its role in health and disease. *J. Mol. Med.* 2004 Jul;82(7):434-48.

[98] Ding GJ, Fischer PA, Boltz RC, Schmidt JA, Colaianne JJ, Gough A, et al. Characterization and quantitation of NF-kappaB nuclear translocation induced by interleukin-1 and tumor necrosis factor-alpha. Development and use of a high capacity fluorescence cytometric system. *J. Biol. Chem.* 1998 Oct 30;273(44):28897-905.

[99] Fujisawa K, Aono H, Hasunuma T, Yamamoto K, Mita S, Nishioka K. Activation of transcription factor NF-kappa B in human synovial cells in response to tumor necrosis factor alpha. *Arthritis Rheum.* 1996 Feb;39(2):197-203.

[100] Calamita G. The Escherichia coli aquaporin-Z water channel. *Mol. Microbiol.* 2000 Jul;37(2):254-62.

[101] Agre P, King LS, Yasui M, Guggino WB, Ottersen OP, Fujiyoshi Y, et al. Aquaporin water channels--from atomic structure to clinical medicine. *J. Physiol.* 2002 Jul 1;542(Pt 1):3-16.

[102] King LS, Kozono D, Agre P. From structure to disease: the evolving tale of aquaporin biology. *Nat. Rev. Mol. Cell Biol.* 2004 Sep;5(9):687-98.

[103] Agre P, Kozono D. Aquaporin water channels: molecular mechanisms for human diseases. *FEBS Lett.* 2003 Nov 27;555(1):72-8.

[104] Schaffner AR. Aquaporin function, structure, and expression: are there more surprises to surface in water relations? *Planta.* 1998 Feb;204(2):131-9.

[105] Chrispeels MJ, Maurel C. Aquaporins: the molecular basis of facilitated water movement through living plant cells? *Plant Physiol.* 1994 May;105(1):9-13.

[106] Johansson I, Karlsson M, Johanson U, Larsson C, Kjellbom P. The role of aquaporins in cellular and whole plant water balance. Biochim *Biophys Acta.* 2000 May 1;1465(1-2):324-42.

[107] Verkman AS, Mitra AK. Structure and function of aquaporin water channels. *Am. J. Physiol. Renal. Physiol.* 2000 Jan;278(1):F13-28.

[108] Verkman AS. Aquaporin water channels and endothelial cell function. *J. Anat.* 2002 Jun;200(6):617-27.

[109] Brown D, Katsura T, Kawashima M, Verkman AS, Sabolic I. Cellular distribution of the aquaporins: a family of water channel proteins. *Histochem. Cell Biol.* 1995 Jul;104(1):1-9.

[110] Castle NA. Aquaporins as targets for drug discovery. *Drug Discov Today.* 2005 Apr 1;10(7):485-93.

[111] Hibuse T, Maeda N, Nagasawa A, Funahashi T. Aquaporins and glycerol metabolism. *Biochim. Biophys Acta.* 2006 Aug;1758(8):1004-11.

[112] Mobasheri A, Marples D. Expression of the AQP-1 water channel in normal human tissues: a semiquantitative study using tissue microarray technology. *Am. J. Physiol. Cell Physiol.* 2004 Mar;286(3):C529-37.

[113] Mobasheri A, Trujillo E, Bell S, Carter SD, Clegg PD, Martin-Vasallo P, et al. Aquaporin water channels AQP1 and AQP3, are expressed in equine articular chondrocytes. *Vet. J.* 2004 Sep;168(2):143-50.

[114] Mobasheri A, Moskaluk CA, Marples D, Shakibaei M. Expression of aquaporin 1 (AQP1) in human synovitis. *Ann. Anat.* 2010 Apr 20;192(2):116-21.

[115] Richardson SM, Knowles R, Marples D, Hoyland JA, Mobasheri A. Aquaporin expression in the human intervertebral disc. *J. Mol. Histol.* 2008 Jun;39(3):303-9.

[116] Mobasheri A, Wray S, Marples D. Distribution of AQP2 and AQP3 water channels in human tissue microarrays. *J. Mol. Histol.* 2005 Feb;36(1-2):1-14.

[117] Sweeney SE, Firestein GS. Rheumatoid arthritis: regulation of synovial inflammation. *Int. J. Biochem. Cell Biol.* 2004 Mar;36(3):372-8.

[118] Holmlund AB, Eriksson L, Reinholt FP. Synovial chondromatosis of the temporomandibular joint: clinical, surgical and histological aspects. *Int. J. Oral Maxillofac Surg.* 2003 Apr;32(2):143-7.

[119] van den Berg WB. Joint inflammation and cartilage destruction may occur uncoupled. *Springer Semin Immunopathol.* 1998;20(1-2):149-64.

[120] Miotla J, Maciewicz R, Kendrew J, Feldmann M, Paleolog E. Treatment with soluble VEGF receptor reduces disease severity in murine collagen-induced arthritis. *Lab Invest.* 2000 Aug;80(8):1195-205.

[121] Hawkins DL, Cargile JL, MacKay RJ, Broome TA, Skelley LA. Effect of tumor necrosis factor antibody on synovial fluid cytokine activities in equine antebrachiocarpal joints injected with endotoxin. *Am. J. Vet. Res.* 1995 Oct;56(10):1292-9.

[122] Mould AW, Tonks ID, Cahill MM, Pettit AR, Thomas R, Hayward NK, et al. Vegfb gene knockout mice display reduced pathology and synovial angiogenesis in both antigen-induced and collagen-induced models of arthritis. *Arthritis Rheum.* 2003 Sep;48(9):2660-9.

[123] Walsh DA, Rodway HA, Claxson A. Vascular turnover during carrageenan synovitis in the rat. *Lab Invest.* 1998 Dec;78(12):1513-21.

[124] Trujillo E, Gonzalez T, Marin R, Martin-Vasallo P, Marples D, Mobasheri A. Human articular chondrocytes, synoviocytes and synovial microvessels express aquaporin water channels; upregulation of AQP1 in rheumatoid arthritis. *Histol. Histopathol.* 2004 Apr;19(2):435-44.

[125] Verkman AS. Role of aquaporin water channels in eye function. *Exp. Eye Res.* 2003 Feb;76(2):137-43.

[126] Virkki LV, Cooper GJ, Boron WF. Cloning and functional expression of an MIP (AQP0) homolog from killifish (Fundulus heteroclitus) lens. *Am. J. Physiol. Regul. Integr. Comp. Physiol.* 2001 Dec;281(6):R1994-2003.

[127] Maunsbach AB, Marples D, Chin E, Ning G, Bondy C, Agre P, et al. Aquaporin-1 water channel expression in human kidney. *J. Am. Soc. Nephrol.* 1997 Jan;8(1):1-14.

[128] Verkman AS. Physiological importance of aquaporins: lessons from knockout mice. *Curr. Opin. Nephrol. Hypertens.* 2000 Sep;9(5):517-22.

[129] Nielsen S, King LS, Christensen BM, Agre P. Aquaporins in complex tissues. II. Subcellular distribution in respiratory and glandular tissues of rat. *Am. J. Physiol.* 1997 Nov;273(5 Pt 1):C1549-61.

In: Arthritis: Types, Treatment and Prevention   ISBN 978-1-61470-719-6
Editor: Marc N. Pelt   © 2012 Nova Science Publishers, Inc.

Chapter IV

Concurrent Treatment of Psoriasis and Psoriatic Arthritis

Emily Yiping Gan, Hong-Liang Tey*
and Wei-Sheng Chong
National Skin Centre, Singapore

ABSTRACT

Psoriasis is a multisystem disease with predominantly skin and joint manifestations, affecting 2% of the population. The proportion of patients with psoriasis who will develop psoriatic arthritis (PsA) ranges from 6% to 42% in different studies.

Not all therapies that target psoriasis however, can successfully treat PsA and vice versa.

The systemic agents – methotrexate, ciclosporin, leflunomide and numerous biologics can treat both skin and joint disease. Methotrexate decreases T and B cell function and suppresses cytokine secretion. Ciclosporin inhibits cytokine promoters with resultant decreased T-cell growth and migration. Leflunomide has both anti-proliferative and anti-inflammatory effects.

Biologics have now been increasingly used for patients with both psoriasis and PsA where first-line therapy has failed. A detailed work-up is necessary prior to initiation.

The first biological agents widely used for psoriasis and PsA are the TNF inhibitors comprising adalimumab, etanercept and infliximab. Adalimumab is the first fully human anti-TNF-α-monoclonal antibody.

Etanercept is a recombinant human TNF-α receptor (p75) protein fused with the Fc portion of IgG1. Infliximab is a chimeric antibody comprising a mouse variable region and human IgG1-α constant region.

Golimumab is a newer monoclonal antibody, which binds to soluble and transmembrane forms of TNF-α. Improvements in PsA and skin disease have been reported in the large phase III multicenter, randomized, placebo-controlled study (Go-REVEAL). Certolizumab pegol (CDP 870) is a pegylated Fab fragment of a humanized anti-TNF-α antibody and in patients with moderate to severe plaque psoriasis, has shown results comparable with adalimumab and infliximab. So far, no phase III studies have been conducted for PsA patients.

Alefacept and efalizumab are T-cell modulators. Alefacept blocks the activation and proliferation of the key T-cells in psoriasis and aids granzyme-mediated apoptosis of T cells. Efalizumab has unfortunately been withdrawn from the market.

Newer agents in the therapeutic armamentarium are the anti-IL-12p40 antibodies: ustekinumab and briakinumab. Ustekinumab is a human immunoglobulin monoclonal antibody to the shared p40 subunit of IL-12 and IL-23. The effect of ustekinumab on cutaneous psoriasis appears to be at least comparable to or better than that of TNF inhibitors and is also promising for PsA. Briakinumab (ABT-874) is a recombinant, fully human IgG1 monoclonal antibody that binds to the same p40 subunit. Early studies have shown high efficacy in the treatment of psoriasis.

This chapter provides an overview of the concurrent treatment strategies for both the skin and joint manifestations of psoriasis.

INTRODUCTION

Psoriasis is a multisystem disease with predominantly skin and joint manifestations, affecting 2-3% of the population [1]. The disease can also affect the heart, aorta and lungs. The proportion of patients with psoriasis who will develop psoriatic arthritis (PsA) remains controversial, ranging from 6% to 42% in different studies. A recent systematic review reported that psoriatic arthritis may affect up to 24% of psoriasis patients [2].

Psoriasis usually appears 8-10 years before PsA [1] although some patients present with PsA sine psoriasis. As both are immune-mediated chronic inflammatory diseases with a similar pathogenesis, concurrent treatment should be undertaken to minimize medication side effects and financial burden [3].

Pathogenesis of Psoriasis and Psoriatic Arthritis Overlaps

With a better understanding of the immune-mediated mechanisms that underlie psoriasis and PsA, new therapies have now been developed to target specific components of the inflammatory pathway. T cell activation is a key part of the process and both the innate and adaptive immune systems are involved. Specifically, T_H1 and T_H17 cells are upregulated in psoriasis lesions [4]. Elevated levels of interferon (IFN)-γ, tumor necrosis factor (TNF)-α and interleukin (IL)-12 are found in psoriasis, providing evidence for the T_H1 pathway [5]. Activated T cells migrate to the dermis where they interact with the dendritic cells and histiocytes causing them to produce IL-12 and IL-23. IL-23, together with TGF-β, IL-6 and IL-21 favors the differentiation of naïve T cells into T_H17 cells with subsequent production of IL-17A, IL-17F, IL-22 and IL-26 IL-17A, IL-17F and IL-22 then act on keratinocytes leading toepidermal hyperplasia, acanthosis and hyperparakeratosis [5,6].

In PsA, similar events occur, with the exception of the activated T cells migrating into the synovium instead of the skin. Studies have confirmed the presence of cytokines including TNF-α, IL-1β, IL-2, IL-10 and IFN-γ in synovial tissue [7], consistent with the cytokine profile in psoriatic lesions. These pro-inflammatory cytokines stimulate production of cellular adhesion molecules with subsequent T cell migration through the vascular endothelium into the synovium, forming leukocytic infiltrates. In the joint, TNF and IL-1 released from activated T cells and mesenchymal cells stimulate synovial proliferation, causing the release of matrix metalloproteinases that can cause joint damage [8].

Choosing the Right Therapy

Selection of therapy for psoriasis must take into account several specific considerations: type of psoriasis, severity and extent of the disease based on the PASI score (Psoriasis Area Severity Index), symptoms such as pain and pruritus, accessibility to ultraviolet light therapy, Dermatology Life Quality Index (DLQI) or other quality of life indices and functional health surveys such as the SF-36 and Health Assessment Questionnaire (HAQ). In PsA, the area of involvement namely peripheral arthritis, axial disease, dactylitis, enthesitis or nail disease influences management decisions. In general, other factors like age of the patient, co-morbidities, response to previous treatment, economic factors and impact on lifestyle also play a role in helping the physician decide the best modality of treatment [9]. Accurate recognition and diagnosis of PsA in the dermatology clinic based on the CASPAR (Classification criteria for Psoriatic Arthritis) criteria [10] together with institution of concurrent treatment of both skin and joint disease, adds to the holistic management of the patient.

Not all therapies that target psoriasis can successfully treat PsA and vice versa. In treating psoriasis alone, commonly used agents include topical corticosteroids, coal tar, vitamin D analogues (e.g. calcipotriol), topical tazarotene, narrow band ultraviolet B (NBUVB) phototherapy, psoralen plus ultraviolet A (PUVA) photochemotherapy and oral retinoids (e.g. acitretin).

For treatment of PsA alone, non-steroidal anti-inflammatory drugs (NSAIDs), intra-articular corticosteroid injections and disease-modifying anti-rheumatic drugs (DMARDs) such as sulfasalazine are the agents commonly prescribed. The physician must be aware that although able to control symptoms, the traditional DMARDs and NSAIDs unfortunately do not retard progression of radiographic joint damage [11], compared to the TNF inhibitors, which are capable of doing so.

There are systemic and biological agents that can target both skin and joints together and these should be prescribed in patients whose disease involves both organs (Table 1). We propose an algorithm for the treatment of patients afflicted with skin and/ or joint disease (Figure 1).

Table 1. List of Drugs that can be used for both Psoriasis and PsA

Systemic agents	Biological agents
Methotrexate	TNF inhibitors: adalimumab, etanercept, infliximab, golimumab, certolizumab
Ciclosporin	T-cell modulators: alefacept
Leflunomide	Anti-IL-12p40: ustekinumab, briakinumab

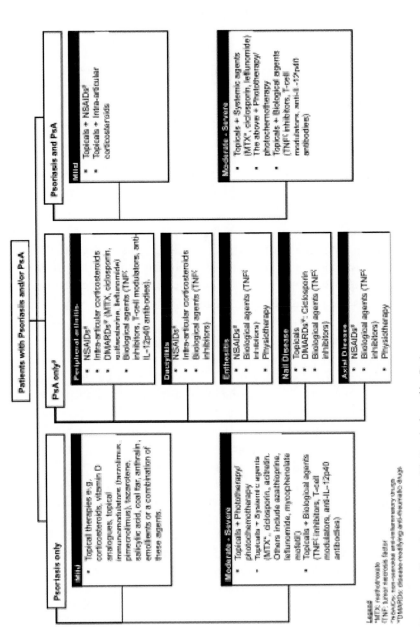

Figure 1. Treatment flow for patients with Psoriasis and/or PsA.

SYSTEMIC AGENTS

Conventional systemic therapies, which have demonstrated effectiveness in both psoriasis and PsA include methotrexate (MTX), ciclosporin (CsA) and leflunomide. The advent of biological agents for the treatment of psoriasis and PsA has not precluded the use of these drugs and they continue to play an important role due to their oral route of administration and lower cost.

1. Methotrexate (MTX)

Mechanism of Action

MTX binds to dihydrofolate reductase to reduce the synthesis of tetrahydrofolate and subsequently purines. This causes decreased DNA synthesis, mitosis inhibition and a reduction in the proliferation of rapidly dividing cells [12]. Besides affecting the cell cycle, MTX also decreases T and B cell functions and suppresses the secretion of cytokines such as IL-1, IFN-γ and TNF-α.

Efficacy

Most studies on the efficacy of MTX performed during the 1960s and 1970s do not comply with the methodological standards applied today. In more recent studies, Heydendael et al compared the efficacy of MTX with ciclosporin in a randomized trial [13]. Using PASI 90 as the endpoint, the study demonstrated that after 16 weeks of treatment, 40% of patients treated with MTX achieved total remission compared to those taking ciclosporin (33%; p=0.55). However, with a PASI reduction of 75%, more patients on ciclosporin (71%) achieved partial remission compared to MTX (60%; p=0.29). Asawananda et al have reported synergism of MTX with NBUVB phototherapy [14]. After 24 weeks, a PASI reduction of 90% was achieved in 91% of patients on both MTX and NBUVB phototherapy, whereas only 38% of patients achieved the same success after NBUVB monotherapy.

Studies on the use of MTX monotherapy in PsA are limited, especially in the era of biological agents. Scarpa et al recently demonstrated that the early use of MTX in patients with early PsA markedly improves tender and swollen joint counts [15]. There was however no significant difference in patient global assessment (PGA), physician's global assessment (PhGA), patient's assessment of pain (VAS), erythrocyte sedimentation rate (ESR) and C-reactive protein (CRP) when compared to the patients for which MTX was initiated later in the course of the disease. Numerous studies, however, support the use of MTX as part of combination systemic therapies for PsA [16]. Drugs that have formed synergistic combination pairs with MTX include ciclosporin [17], alefacept [18] and ustekinumab [19]. MTX-TNF inhibitors(etanercept, infliximab, adalimumab or golimumab) combinations have all not been shown to improve clinical efficacy in PsA when compared to the biological agent alone [16].

The Group for Research and Assessment of Psoriasis and Psoriatic Arthritis (GRAPPA) has recommended the use of MTX in patients with peripheral arthritis and skin disease but not axial disease, dactylitis or enthesitis in PsA [9].

Dosage

MTX is given once weekly and can be administered via oral or parenteral routes (intramuscular or subcutaneous injections). For the oral drug, it is possible to split the dose into 3 separate doses at 12-hour intervals over a 24-hour period. This reduces risks of gastrointestinal adverse effects [20]. Test doses of 2.5mg or 5mg are usually given and the doses increased according to response. Complete clinical responses may take several weeks to manifest. In the elderly or those with renal impairment, caution should be exercised with MTX as its primary route of excretion is via the kidneys.

Drug Interactions

MTX has potential for drug interactions with numerous drugs. Decreased renal elimination of MTX can occur with concurrent use of colchicine, ciclosporin, penicillin, NSAIDs and salicylates; increased risk of bone marrow and gastrointestinal toxicity occurs with NSAIDs and antibiotics such as chloramphenicol and co-trimoxazole; increased hepatotoxicty results with simultaneous use of leflunomide, retinoids, tetracyclines and ethanol; lastly, interaction with plasma protein binding occurs with use of barbiturates, NSAIDs, co-trimoxazole, phenytoin and probenecid [21].

Adverse Drug Reactions/ Toxicity

Most frequent side effects are nausea, malaise and hair loss. Other adverse reactions in order of decreasing frequency are elevated transaminases, bone marrow suppression, gastrointestinal ulcers, infection, liver fibrosis, interstitial pneumonitis and alveolitis [21]. Exposure to high levels of MTX in combination with PUVA is an independent risk factor for the development of squamous cell carcinoma [22].

Risk of liver fibrosis or cirrhosis is minimal if appropriate screening measures and monitoring procedures are followed. Risk factors for hepatotoxicity include patients with diabetes mellitus, obesity, the metabolic syndrome, nonalcoholic steatohepatitis [23,24], patients who have a cumulative intake of more than 3.5-4.0g of MTX [25] and alcohol consumption of more than 100g per week [26].

Drug Monitoring

Recently released guidelines from the National Psoriasis Foundation recommend that patients should be monitored regularly with laboratory tests (Table 2) [27]. A significant reduction in leukocyte or platelet count warrants reduction or temporary discontinuation of MTX. Rescue therapy with folinic acid can be considered for cases with clinically significant leukopenia or thrombocytopenia. Increasing mean corpuscular volume suggests developing macrocytic anemia. Folic acid supplementation administered orally in dosages of 1-5 mg daily may prevent or reverse this side effect. Oral folinic acid supplementation is an alternative. Patients at risk of hematologic toxicity will require more frequent monitoring.

Table 2. Continuing Laboratory Tests for Methotrexate therapy

Laboratory Test	Timing of Test
Complete blood count	After 7-14 days: when starting therapy or after an increase in dose Every 2-4 weeks: first few months of therapy Every 1-3 months: when patient is on a stable dose
Renal function studies	Every 2-3 months: serum creatinine and blood urea nitrogen
Liver chemistries	Every 4-12 weeks: ALT (alanine aminotransferase), AST (aspartate aminotransferase), ALP (alkaline phosphatase) and serum albumin levels
Pregnancy Test	If indicated, in women of child-bearing potential

From the management point of view, patients should be divided into 2 groups – those with metabolic risk factors for hepatotoxicity and those without. Patients in the latter group should be judged by the American College of Rheumatology Criteria for monitoring MTX, which has been validated in patients with rheumatoid arthritis and has resulted in a decrease in the number of liver biopsies [28]. These criteria include an evaluation of liver chemistries every 1-3 months with a need for liver biopsy only if 5 of 9 aspartate aminotransferase (AST) levels are elevated during a 12-month period or if there is a reduction in albumin level below normal in a patient with well-controlled disease. In addition, a cumulative dose of MTX of 3.5-4.0g has been shown to be a more appropriate time frame for the first liver biopsy in patients without preexisting risk factors for hepatotoxicity [29].

In patients with risk factors for hepatotoxicity, consideration should be given to the use of a different systemic agent, performance of a delayed baseline liver biopsy and repeated liver biopsies after approximately 1-1.5g of MTX [27]. A delayed baseline liver biopsy should be carried out only 2-6 months after starting MTX as the medication may be discontinued within this initial period in patients who suffer adverse effects or who show a lack of clinical effectiveness.

2. Ciclosporin

Mechanism of Action

The immunosuppressive effects of ciclosporin arise from its binding with the immunosuppressant-binding protein cyclophilin. This process inhibits cytokine promoters, leading to reduction in transcription and processing of cytokines (IL-2 and IFN-γ) within T cells, eventually resulting in decreased T cell growth and migration [12].

Efficacy

Multiple studies support the efficacy of ciclosporin and when given at 2.5-5 mg/kg/day for 12-16 weeks, rapid and dramatic improvement occurs in up to 80-90% of psoriasis patients [30-32]. Short-term treatment with ciclosporin is a good option as toxicity risks are reduced and it is generally well tolerated. Long-term ciclosporin use in psoriasis has also been reported. Mrowietz et al studied 217 patients who were treated for 6-30 months with ciclosporin at 1.25, 2.5 or 5.0 mg/kg/day and 12.5% of patients were successfully maintained on 1.25 mg/kg/day without loss of efficacy [33]. In another study, 142 patients with severe psoriasis, who responded to an induction phase of ciclosporin treatment, were continued on a 6-month maintenance regime at 3mg/kg/day. At 6 months, only 42% of those in the maintenance arm had suffered a relapse compared to 84% of those on placebo [34].

The drug is primarily indicated for induction therapy in adults with moderate to severe psoriasis, who do not respond sufficiently to topical therapy and/ or phototherapy. It can be considered for long-term therapy (up to 2 years) on a case-by-case basis but patients need to be closely monitored for adverse effects [21].

Similar to MTX, GRAPPA has recommended the use of ciclosporin in patients with peripheral arthritis and skin disease but not axial disease, dactylitis or enthesitis in PsA [9]. When used with MTX, ciclosporin is synergistic in improving PsA treatment outcomes [17]. However, the additive immunosuppressive effect increases the risk of infection and carcinogenesis and the use of the combination for prolonged periods should be avoided.

Dosage

The initial dose of ciclosporin is 2.5-3 mg/kg/day in 2 divided doses. This dose is maintained for 4 weeks and then increased at increments of 0.5 mg/kg/day until disease control is achieved. The maximum dose for psoriasis is typically 5 mg/kg/day [25]. Short-term therapy over 8-16 weeks with dose reduction at the end of the period or continuous long-term therapy up to a maximum of 2 years can be undertaken. In the latter, after achieving disease control, dose reduction should occur every 2 weeks until a maintenance dosage of 0.5-3 mg/kg/day [21]. Administration of ciclosporin should occur at a consistent time of the day so as to reduce intra-individual blood level variations.

Drug Interactions

Ciclosporin is metabolized by the cytochrome P450 3A4 system. Drugs that increase ciclosporin levels include macrolides, fluoroquinolones, sertraline, statins, losartan, calcium channel blockers like diltiazem and nifedipine and antifungals like fluconazole, itraconazole and ketoconazole. On the other hand, rifampicin, griseofulvin, anticonvulsants like carbamazepine, phenytoin, phenobarbital and valproic acid among others, will decrease ciclosporin levels.

Ciclosporin also inhibits P-glycoprotein (P-gp), an efflux transporter which pumps drugs out of cells like enterocytes and renal epithelial cells. Therefore, when prescribed together with P-gp substrates such as digoxin, it increases the substrate's bioavailability by increasing intestinal absorption and reducing renal elimination [35].

Increased risk of nephrotoxic adverse drug reaction occurs when there is concomitant use of aminoglycosides like gentamicin, amphotericin B, NSAIDs and vancomycin. It is thus recommended that the creatinine values be checked more frequently when prescribing both these drugs and ciclosporin.

Adverse Drug Reactions/ Toxicity

The adverse effects of ciclosporin are dose dependent [36]. The most frequently reported adverse effect is on the kidney and blood pressure. An increase in serum creatinine of 5-30% with a reduced creatinine clearance up to an average of 20%, has been reported.

Arterial hypertension occurs in 2-15% of patients [21]. Gastrointestinal symptoms such as nausea, diarrhea and flatulence occur in 10-30% of patients and gingival hyperplasia in up to 15%. Other side effects include hypertrichosis, hyperuricemia, hypomagnesemia, hyperglycaemia, hyperlipidemia and headaches [21]. There is also an increased risk of various bacterial, parasitic, viral and fungal infections and infections with opportunistic pathogens.

Being an immunosuppressant, ciclosporin increases the risk of malignancies, especially lymphoproliferative disorders and skin cancers, a phenomenon that is well documented among organ transplant recipients [37]. In psoriasis patients who were treated with ciclosporin, Paul et al reported the incidence of malignancies to be twice the rate of the general population [38].

This was in part attributable to a 6-fold greater risk of non melanoma skin cancer, with the majority being squamous cell carcinoma. The incidence of non-cutaneous malignancies including lymphoproliferative disorders, was however not significantly higher than the general population. Addition of PUVA photochemotherapy to the treatment regime increases the incidence of malignancies further.

Marcil et al studied a cohort of patients who were previously on PUVA therapy and reported a 7 times greater risk of squamous cell carcinoma after commencing ciclosporin, compared to that seen in the 5 years prior to ciclosporin usage [39].

Drug Monitoring

Patients should be monitored every other week with blood pressure readings, serum creatinine, blood urea nitrogen and a complete blood count for the first 3 months and subsequently at monthly intervals. Other laboratory tests include urinalysis 4 weeks after initiation and then 12 weeks later, as well as fasting lipids every 8 weeks [21].

3. Leflunomide

Mechanism of Action

Leflunomide has both anti-proliferative and anti-inflammatory effects. It inhibits de novo synthesis of pyrimidines. As activated lymphocytes require a large pyrimidine pool, leflunomide preferentially inhibits T cell activation and proliferation [40].

Efficacy

Small open-label trials have demonstrated efficacy of leflunomide in causing an improvement in both joint and skin symptoms [41,42]. The Treatment of Psoriatic Arthritis Study (TOPAS) was a large randomized, double-blind placebo-controlled, multinational trial of 190 patients with both psoriasis and PsA [43]. After 24 weeks, 58.9% of leflunomide-treated patients were classified as responders according to the Psoriatic Arthritis Response Criteria compared to 29.7% of placebo-treated patients. Using the PASI 50 as an outcome measure, 30.4% of leflunomide-treated patients achieved the target compared to 18.9% of placebo-treated patients, a result which reached statistical significance. Quality of life evaluations also showed significant improvements in the leflunomide group in terms of the DLQI, HAQ and SF-36 scores [44].

Dosage

In the TOPAS study, a loading dose of 100mg of leflunomide was administered orally once daily for 3 days with subsequently daily dose of 20mg [43].

Drug Interactions

This is not as significant as MTX and ciclosporin. If given together with methotrexate, there is an increased risk of hepatotoxicity [25].

Adverse Drug Reactions/ Toxicity

Adverse effects associated with leflunomide are predominantly gastrointestinal including diarrhea, nausea, dyspepsia, elevated liver enzymes, leucopenia, drug eruption, headaches and increased risk of infections [45].

Drug Monitoring

Monthly complete blood count and liver function tests, including aminotransferases should be done for the first 6 months and every 6-8 weeks thereafter [25].

BIOLOGICAL AGENTS

Biologics have now been increasingly used for patients with both psoriasis and PsA when first-line therapy has failed. A detailed work-up including history, physical examination, relevant laboratory and radiological investigations is necessary prior to the commencement of biologics. The Medical Board of the National Psoriasis Foundation recently released a consensus statement recommending that screening tests including complete blood count, liver function tests, hepatitis panel and tuberculosis testing be carried out at baseline and at intervals thereafter. While on therapy, patients should be periodically re-evaluated for new symptoms suggestive of infection or malignancy.

Vaccination with live vaccines such as yellow fever or live-attenuated vaccines like varicella, MMR (measles, mumps and rubella) or intranasal influenza, should be avoided in patients on immunosuppressive therapy. It is preferable to obtain these vaccinations prior to initiation of biologic therapy [46].

1. TNF Inhibitors – Adalimumab, Etanercept, Infliximab, Golimumab

The first biological agents widely used for psoriasis and PsA are the TNF inhibitors consisting of adalimumab, etanercept and infliximab. All have been shown to improve both skin and joint disease. Newer drugs in this category include golimumab and certolizumab. In general, patients who fail 1 TNF inhibitor due to a side effect may be expected to have a better clinical response compared to patients who fail due to loss of efficacy [47].

There have been more than 50 reports since 2005, on the paradoxical development of psoriasis and psoriasiform lesions, mainly plaque psoriasis and palmoplantar pustulosis, following the use of TNF inhibitors such as adalimumab, etanercept, infliximab [48] and certolizumab [49,50] in the treatment of patients with rheumatoid arthritis or inflammatory bowel disease. One postulated mechanism for this occurrence is that of cytokine imbalance, with decreased TNF-α and increased IFN-α levels, which activates dendritic cells leading to increased antigen presentation in the skin. Other possible mechanisms include an enhancement of the chemokine receptor CXR3 leading to upregulation in psoriasis lesions and promotion of autoreactive T cell infiltration in the skin [51]; a change in T cell function or an immune allergic reaction [48]. Increased awareness of this adverse effect of TNF inhibitors is important and further studies are needed to clarify the underlying mechanism.

(a) Adalimumab (Humira ®)

Adalimumab is the first fully human anti-TNF-α-monoclonal antibody and it binds specifically to soluble and membrane-bound TNF-α, blocking TNF-α interactions with the p55 and p75 cell surface TNF receptors.

Gordon et al reported on the first dose-ranging, double-blind, randomized controlled trial and extension study for the use of adalimumab in moderate to severe chronic plaque-type psoriasis [52]. The adalimumab treatment groups received subcutaneous injections of adalimumab 80mg at week 0 prior to initiating every other week or weekly dosing at week 1, continuing for an additional 48 weeks. By week 12, 53% of patients in the every other week arm and 80% of patients in the weekly arm achieved PASI 75, significantly more than the 4% of the patients in the placebo group. Good clinical response was sustained for 60 weeks.

More recently, Menter et al conducted a 52-week multicenter, multiphase study of 1212 patients randomized to receive subcutaneous injections of adalimumab 40mg or placebo every other week for the first 15 weeks, with advancement into the subsequent phase of maintenance treatment only for responders (PASI 75) at week 16 and a re-randomization for responders at week 33. At week 16, 71% of adalimumab-treated patients compared to 7% of placebo-treated patients advanced to the 2nd phase of the study. At week 52,

28% of patients who were re-randomized to placebo lost adequate response compared to just 5% of those who had been on continuous adalimumab [53].

In PsA, Mease et al conducted the Adalimumab Effectiveness in Psoriatic Arthritis Trial (ADEPT), the first double-blind, randomized, placebo-controlled trial of adalimumab for patients with moderate to severe active PsA and a history of inadequate response to NSAIDs [54]. A total of 315 patients were randomized to receive 40mg of adalimumab or placebo subcutaneously every other week for 24 weeks. At week 24, 57% of the adalimumab-treated patients achieved ACR 20 (20% improvement in the American College of Rheumatology criteria), compared to 15% of the placebo-treated patients (p<0.001). For skin disease, 59% achieved a PASI 75 score at 24 weeks, compared with 1% in the placebo arm (p<0.001).

Gladman et al conducted an open label study to evaluate the efficacy and safety of adalimumab treatment over 48 weeks in 151 patients with moderate to severe PsA, who had completed the adalimumab arm of the ADEPT study [55]. These patients were treated with adalimumab 40mg subcutaneously every other week for up to 120 weeks. There were improved joint and skin manifestations, reduced disability and inhibited radiographic progression over 48 weeks, together with a good safety profile.

The recommended dosing schedule for psoriasis is subcutaneous injections of 80mg in the first week, 40mg in the 2nd week and then 40mg every other week [46]. For PsA, subcutaneous injections of 40mg every other week is recommended [56].

(b) Etanercept (Enbrel ®)

Etanercept consists of a recombinant human TNF-α receptor (p75) protein fused with the Fc portion of IgG1 and it binds to soluble and membrane-bound TNF-α.

The efficacy of etanercept in the treatment of psoriasis has been shown in many trials [57-59]. In one such study by Leonardi et al, after 12 weeks, an improvement of PASI 75 or more was demonstrated in 34% of etanercept-treated patients receiving 25mg twice weekly and 49% of those receiving 50mg twice weekly compared to 4% in the placebo group (p<0.001). The reduction in severity of disease was maintained at 24 weeks [59].

In a phase III study of 205 PsA patients, Mease et al demonstrated significant improvement in PsA with etanercept administered at 25mg twice weekly [60]. Tender and swollen joints counts, morning stiffness, C-reactive protein levels and physician and patient global ratings all improved significantly compared to placebo. Radiologic disease progression was also inhibited in the etanercept-treated group.

The recommended dosing schedule for psoriasis is subcutaneous injections of 50mg twice a week for 3 months followed by 50mg weekly [46]. For PsA, subcutaneous injections of 25mg twice a week or 50mg weekly is recommended [56].

(c) Infliximab (Remicade ®)

Infliximab is a chimeric antibody made from murine and human DNA sequences comprising a mouse variable region and a human IgG1-α constant region. It binds with high avidity, affinity and specificity to TNF-α. By antagonizing TNF-α, infliximab is believed to reduce the upregulation of adhesion molecules on endothelial cells, the vascular changes seen in psoriasis, the release of pro-inflammatory cytokines from antigen presenting cells and T cells, keratinocyte proliferation and synovial tissue damage [61].

Numerous trials have proven the efficacy of infliximab in treating both psoriasis [62-64] and PsA [65,66]. Amongst them, the Infliximab Multinational Psoriatic Arthritis Controlled Trial (IMPACT) was a 2-phase, double-blind, placebo-controlled randomized study analyzing the effect of infliximab infusion on PsA and psoriasis [65]. At week 16, 65% of infliximab-treated patients achieved an ACR 20 response compared to 10% of those in the placebo arm (p<0.001). None of the placebo-treated patients achieved more than 75% improvement in PASI score at week 16 compared to 68% of infliximab-treated patients (p<0.001). The improvement was sustained through 50 weeks of treatment.

The recommended dosing schedules are the same for both psoriasis and PsA: 5mg/kg dose infusion schedule at weeks 0, 2, 6 and 6-8 weekly subsequently, adjusted according to requirement [46,56].

Human antichimeric antibodies (HACA) to infliximab are less likely to develop and clinical responses are better maintained if patients are treated continuously rather than on an as-needed, intermittent basis [62,63]. Combination of infliximab with immunosuppressants such as MTX at a maintenance dose of 15mg weekly, has been shown to suppress antibody formation [67] and hence reduce the rate of infliximab-related infusion reactions in patients with Crohn's disease and rheumatoid arthritis [68]. Unfortunately, there are no such studies in psoriasis patients. Based on the same theory of reduction of antibody development, Pathirana et al suggests combining low-dose MTX with infliximab to maintain clinical efficacy over time [21].

(d) Golimumab (Simponi ®)

Golimumab is a very promising newer monoclonal antibody, which binds with high specificity and affinity to the soluble and transmembrane forms of TNF-α [69].

Improvements in PsA and skin disease have been reported in a large phase III multicenter, randomized, placebo-controlled study (Go-REVEAL) [70]. This study involved 405 patients who were enrolled at 58 sites. Patients were randomized to injections of 50mg, 100mg or placebo every 4 weeks and were allowed stable doses of MTX up to 25mg/ week. At week 14, 40% of the 50mg group and 58% of the 100mg group achieved PASI 75, compared to 3% in the placebo group (p<0.001). Signs and symptoms of PsA also improved significantly. At week 14, 51% and 45% of patients in the 50mg and 100mg groups respectively, attained an ACR 20 response compared to 9% in the placebo group (p<0.001). The efficacy of the drug on skin and joint manifestations was maintained through week 24. Significant improvement was also seen in the golimumab group for other endpoints such as the SF-36 and HAQ scores.

(e) Certolizumab (Cimzia ®)

Certolizumab pegol (CDP 870) is another newer TNF inhibitor. It is a pegylated Fab fragment of a humanized anti-TNF-α antibody. It binds to TNF-α, inhibiting its interaction with cell surface receptors. Approval has been obtained for use in rheumatoid arthritis and inflammatory bowel disease in several countries but there have been limited published studies in psoriasis.

Ortonne et al reported preliminary results of a phase II trial where patients were randomized to receive subcutaneous certolizumab pegol 200mg, 400mg or placebo every 2 weeks up to week 12 [71]. Significantly more patients receiving certolizumab pegol 200mg or 400mg achieved PASI 75 compared to the placebo group by week 12 (74.6% and 82.8% versus 6.8%). The PASI 75 results and side effects were comparable to the other TNF inhibitors adalimumab and infliximab. So far, no phase III studies or studies in PsA patients have been published, however, it is expected to have similar results compared to other TNF inhibitors.

2. T-Cell Modulators – Alefacept, Efalizumab

Alefacept was the first biological agent approved by the Food and Drug Administration in the United States for the treatment of psoriasis [72] and is currently the only drug in this class. Efalizumab, a humanized monoclonal antibody directed against lymphocyte function associated antigen-1 (LFA-1), was withdrawn from the market in 2009 after reports of progressive multifocal leukoencephalopathy in patients on long-term treatment [73].

(a) Alefacept (Amevive ®)

Alefacept is a recombinant human LFA-3 IgG1 fusion protein. It inhibits T cell activation and proliferation and causes T cell apoptosis, resulting in a selective decrease in effector memory T cells and modification of the inflammatory process in psoriasis [21].

In a multicenter, randomized, double-blind study, patients who received 12 weeks of once-weekly 0.075mg/kg of intravenous alefacept achieved a 53% reduction in the mean PASI score compared to a 21% reduction in the placebo group (p<0.001) [74]. In another study, 21% of patients had at least a PASI 75 response when given 15mg of intramuscular alefacept once weekly, compared to 5% in the placebo group (p<0.001) [75]. Patients with at least a PASI 75 response to a 12-week course of alefacept managed to maintain at least a PASI 50 response for a median duration of more than 7 months after treatment, highlighting the sustainablility of the drug's effects [76].

Alefacept has modest effects on joint disease. A 12-week controlled, double-blind, phase 2 clinical trial comparing intramuscular alefacept combined with methotrexate against methotrexate alone reported a significant outcome: 54% of 185 patients with active PsA in the former group achieved an ACR 20 response compared to 23% in the latter [18]. An open label extension of the same study, however, concluded that alefacept is less potent than TNF inhibitors [77].

The recommended dosing schedule for psoriasis is 15mg intramuscularly once weekly for 12 weeks. A minimum of 12 weeks is needed between each 12-week course [21].

3. Anti-IL-12p40 Antibodies – Ustekinumab, Briakinumab

Newer agents in the therapeutic armamentarium are the anti-IL-12p40 antibodies – ustekinumab and briakinumab.

(a) Ustekinumab (Stelara ®)

Ustekinumab is a human immunoglobulin IgG1κ monoclonal antibody that binds strongly with the shared p40 subunit of both IL-12 and IL-23. This inhibits binding to IL-12Rβ1 on T-cells, natural killer cells and antigen presenting cells, resulting in a rapid downregulation of T_H1 cytokines, chemokines and IL-12/IL-23 [78].

PHOENIX 1 was a phase III trial conducted in 766 patients to establish the efficacy and safety of ustekinumab in the treatment of psoriasis [79]. Patients received either 45mg of ustekinumab, 90mg of ustekinumab or placebo subcutaneously at weeks 0, 4 and every 12 weeks thereafter. At week 12, PASI 75 was achieved in 67% of those in the 45mg group and 66% of those in the 90mg group, a significantly larger proportion compared to the 3% in the placebo group. At week 40, the patients were re-randomized to either placebo or 12-weekly ustekinumab at their original dose, up to week 76. Those in the former group had a gradual recurrence of disease but no episodes of rebound flare. The patients in the latter group, however, were able to maintain a PASI 75 response for at least a year.

PHOENIX 2 was a larger phase III trial comprising 1230 patients, who were randomized to receive either ustekinumab 45mg, 90mg or placebo at weeks 0, 4 and every 12 weeks thereafter [80]. At week 52, partial responders were re-randomized to either receiving the same or a more frequent dosing schedule. The study concluded that increasing the dosing frequency in partial responders in the 90mg group from every 12 weeks to every 8 weeks resulted in improvement and this was not seen in the 45mg group.

Gottlieb et al reported on a phase II multicenter, randomized, placebo-controlled trial in which PsA patients were randomized to either ustekinumab (63mg or 90mg) every week for 4 weeks followed by placebo at weeks 12 and 16, or placebo for the first 4 weeks followed by ustekinumab (63mg) at weeks 12 and 16 [19]. At week 12, 42% of patients in the ustekinumab arm achieved ACR 20 compared to 14% in the placebo group. The authors concluded that ustekinumab significantly reduces signs and symptoms of psoriatic arthritis and is well tolerated.

The effects of ustekinumab on psoriasis and psoriatic arthritis are promising and more trials are needed to corroborate this.

(b) Briakinumab (Ozespa ®)

Briakinumab (ABT-874) is a more recently introduced recombinant, fully human IgG1 monoclonal antibody that binds to the p40 subunit shared by IL-12 and IL-23. It has so far only been evaluated at the phase II level but the efficacy results are among the highest, if not the highest, of any placebo-controlled trial on the treatment of psoriasis so far [81]. Patients were randomized into 6 groups: to receive either only 1 dose of briakinumab 200mg at week 0, 100mg briakinumab every other week for 12 weeks, 200mg weekly for 4 weeks, 200mg every other week for 12 weeks, 200mg weekly for 12 weeks or placebo (p<0.001). By week 12, a PASI 75 response was achieved in 90% of subjects in all 5 briakinumab groups compared to only 3% in the placebo group. More studies are needed to evaluate this biological agent further, especially on its use in patients with PsA.

CONCLUSION

The approach to the concurrent treatment of psoriasis and PsA requires a good clinical assessment of both conditions and the joint selection of the most appropriate therapy. With the rapid development of new pharmacological therapies, it is imperative for dermatologists to be aware of and to discuss with patients the risks versus benefits prior to initiation of any treatment.

REFERENCES

[1]   Feletar M, Foley P, Brown MA. Developments in psoriasis and psoriatic arthritis. *Drug Discov. Today Dis. Mech.* 2008;5:e47-54.

[2]   Prey S, Paul C, Bronsard V, et al. Assessment of risk of psoriatic arthritis in patients with plaque psoriasis: a systematic review of the literature. *J. Eur. Acad. Dermatol. Venereol* 2010;24:31-5.

[3]   Rapp SR, Feldman SR, Exum L, et al. Psoriasis causes as much disability as other major medical diseases. *J. Am. Acad. Dermatol* 1999;41:401-7.

[4]   Kagami S, Rizzo HL, Lee JJ, et al. Circulating Th17, Th22, and Th1 Cells Are Increased in Psoriasis. *J. Invest Dermatol.* 2010;130:1373-83.

[5]   Di Cesare A, Di Meglio P, Nestle FO. The IL-23/Th17 Axis in the Immunopathogenesis of Psoriasis. *J. Invest Dermatol.* 2009;129:1339-50.

[6]   Sanchez AP. Immunopathogenesis of psoriasis. *An Bras. Dermatol.* 2010;85:747-9.

[7]   Ruderman EM. Evaluation and management of psoriatic arthritis: the role of biologic therapy. *J. Am. Acad. Dermatol.* 2003;49:S125-32.

[8]   Fisher VS. Clinical Monograph for Drug Formulary Review: Systemic Agents for Psoriasis/ Psoriatic Arthritis. *J. Manag. Care Pharm.* 2005;11:33-55.

[9]   Ritchlin CT, Kavanaugh A, Gladman DD. Treatment recommendations for psoriatic arthritis. *Ann. Rheum. Dis.* 2009;68:1387-94.

[10]   Taylor W, Gladman D, Helliwell P, et al. Classification criteria for psoriatic arthritis: development of new criteria from a large international study. *Arthritis Rheum.* 2006;54:2665-73.

[11]   Gladman DD. Traditional and Newer Therapeutic Options for Psoriatic Arthritis. *Drugs* 2005;65:1223-38.

[12]   Yamauchi PS, Rizk D, Kormeili T, et al. Current systemic therapies for psoriasis: where are we now? *J. Am. Acad. Dermatol.* 2003;49:S66-77.

[13]   Heydendael VM, Spuls PI, Opmeer BC, et al. Methotrexate versus cyclosporine in moderate-to-severe chronic plaque psoriasis. *N .Engl. J. Med.* 2003;349:658-65.

[14]   Asawanonda P, Nateetongrungsak Y. Methotrexate plus narrowband UVB phototherapy versus narrowband UVB phototherapy alone in the treatment of plaque-type psoriasis: a randomized, placebo-controlled study. *J. Am. Acad. Dermatol.* 2006;54:1013-8.

[15]   Scarpa R, Peluso R, Atteno M, et al. The effectiveness of a traditional therapeutic approach in early psoriatic arthritis: Results of a pilot randomised 6-month trial with methotrexate. *Clin. Rheumatol.* 2008;27:823-6.

[16]   Daly M, Alikhan A, Armstrong AW. Combination systemic therapies in psoriatic arthritis. *J. Dermatol. Treat.* 2010 Jul 28 [Epub ahead of print].

[17]   Fraser AD, van Kuijk AW, Westhovens R, et al. A randomised, double blind, placebo controlled, multicentre trial of combination therapy with methotrexate plus ciclosporin in patients with active psoriatic arthritis. *Ann. Rheum. Dis.* 2005;64:859-64.

[18]   Mease PJ, Gladman DD, Keystone EC. Alefacept in combination with methotrexate for treatment of psoriatic arthritis: Results of a randomized, double-blind, placebo-controlled study. *Arthritis Rheum.* 2006;54:1638-45.

[19]   Gottlieb A, Menter A, Mendelsohn A, et al. Ustekinumab, a human interleukin 12/23 monoclonal antibody, for psoriatic arthritis: Randomised, double-blind, placebo-controlled, crossover trial. *Lancet* 2009;373:633-40.

[20] Weinstein GD, Frost P. Methotrexate for psoriasis. A new therapeutic schedule. *Arch. Dermatol.* 1971;103:33-8.

[21] Pathirana D, Ormerod AD, Saiag P, et al. European S3-guidelines on the systemic treatment of psoriasis vulgaris. *J. Eur. Acad. Dermatol. Venereol* 2009;23:5-70.

[22] Stern RS. Lymphoma risk in psoriasis. *Arch. Dermatol.* 2006;142:1132-5.

[23] Langman G, Hall PM, Todd G. Role of non-alcoholic steatohepatitis in methotrexate-induced liver injury. *J. Gastroenterol. Hepatol.* 2001;16:1395-401.

[24] Rosenberg P, Urwitz H, Johannesson A, et al. Psoriasis patients with diabetes type 2 are at high risk of developing liver fibrosis during methotrexate treatment. *J. Hepatol.* 2007;46:1111-8.

[25] Menter A, Korman NJ, Elmets CA, et al. Guidelines of care for the management of psoriasis and psoriatic arthritis: Section 4. Guidelines of care for the management and treatment of psoriasis with traditional systemic agents. *J. Am. Acad. Dermatol.* 2009;61:451-85.

[26] Whiting-O'Keefe QE, Fye KH, Sack KD. Methotrexate and histologic hepatic abnormalities: a meta-analysis. *Am. J. Med.* 1991;90:711-6.

[27] Kalb Re, Strober B, Weinstein G, et al. Methotrexate and psoriasis: 2009 National Psoriasis Foundation consensus conference. *J. Am. Acad. Dermatol* 2009;60:824-37.

[28] Erickson AR, Reddy V, Vogelgesang SA, et al. Usefulness of the American College of Rheumatology recommendations for liver biopsy in methotrexate-treated rheumatoid arthritis patients. *Arthritis Rheum.* 1995;38:1115-9.

[29] Thomas JA, Aithal GP. Monitoring liver function during methotrexate therapy for psoriasis: are routine biopsies really necessary? *Am. J. Clin. Dermatol.* 2005;6:357-63.

[30] Berth-Jones J, Henderson CA, Munro CS, et al. Treatment of psoriasis with intermittent short course cyclosporine (Neoral): a multicenter study. *Br. J. Dermatol.* 1997;136:527-30.

[31] Ho VC, Griffiths CE, Albrecht G, et al. Intermittent short courses of cyclosporine (Neoral®) for psoriasis unresponsive to topical therapy: a 1-year multicenter, randomized study; the PISCES study group. *Br. J. Dermatol.* 1999;141:283-91.

[32] Faerber L, Braeutigam M, Weidinger G, et al. Cyclosporine in severe psoriasis: results of a meta-analysis in 579 patients. *Am. J. Clin. Dermatol.* 2001;2:41-7.

[33] Mrowietz U, Farber L, Henneicke-von Zepelin HH, et al. Long-term maintenance therapy with cyclosporine and posttreatment survey in severe psoriasis: results of a multicenter study; German multicenter study. *J. Am. Acad. Dermatol.* 1995;33:470-5.

[34] Shupack J, Abel E, Bauer E, et al. Cyclosporine as maintenance therapy in patients with severe psoriasis. *J. Am. Acad. Dermatol.* 1997;36:423-32.

[35] Smit JW, Duin E, Steen H, et al. Interactions between P-glycoprotein substrates and other cationic drugs at the hepatic excretory level. *Br. J. Clin. Pharmacol.* 1998;123:361-70.

[36] Ellis CN, Fradin MS, Messana JM, et al. Cyclosporine for plaque-type psoriasis. Results of a multidose, multi-blind trial. *N. Engl. J. Med.* 1991;324:277-84.

[37] Cockburn ITR, Krupp P. The Risk of Neoplasms in Patients Treated with Cyclosporine A. *J. Autoimmun.* 1989;2:723-31

[38] Paul CF, Ho VC, McGeown C, et al. Risk of malignancies in psoriasis patients treated with cyclosporine: a 5y cohort study. *J. Invest. Dermatol.* 2003;120:211-6.

[39] Marcil I, Stern RS. Squamous-cell cancer of the skin in patients given PUVA and ciclosporin: nested cohort crossover study. *Lancet* 2001;358:1042-5.

[40] Breedveld FC, Dayer JM. Leflunomide: mode of action in the treatment of rheumatoid arthritis. *Ann Rheum Dis* 2000;59:841-9.

[41] Liang GC, Barr WG. Open trial of leflunomide for refractory psoriasis and psoriatic arthritis. *J Clin Rheumatol* 2001;7:366-70.

[42] Reich K, Hummel KM, Beckman I, et al. Treatment of severe psoriasis and psoriatic arthritis with leflunomide. *Br J Dermatol* 2002;146:335-6.

[43] Kaltwasser JP, Nash P, Gladman D, et al. Efficacy and safety of leflunomide in the treatment of psoriatic arthritis and psoriasis. *Arthritis Rheum* 2004;50:1939-50.

[44] Nash P, Thaci D, Behrens F, et al. Leflunomide improves psoriasis in patients with psoriatic arthritis: an in-depth analysis of data from the TOPAS study. *Dermatology* 2006;212:238-49.

[45] Prakash A, Jarvis B. Leflunomide: a review of its use in active rheumatoid arthritis. *Drugs* 1999;58:1137-64.

[46] Menter A, Gottlieb A, Feldman SR, et al. Guidelines of care for the management of psoriasis and psoriatic arthritis: Section 1. Overview of psoriasis and guidelines of care for the treatment of psoriasis with biologics. *J. Am. Acad. Dermatol.* 2008;58:826-50.

[47] Conti F, Ceccarelli F, Marocchi E, et al. Switching tumour necrosis factor alpha antagonists in patients with ankylosing spondylitis and psoriatic arthritis: An observational study over a 5-year period. *Ann. Rheum Dis* 2007;66:1393-7.

[48] Grinblat B, Scheinberg M. The enigmatic development of psoriasis and psoriasiform lesions during anti-TNF therapy: a review. *Semin. Arthritis Rheum.* 2008;37:251-5.

[49] Mocciaro F, Renna S, Orlando A, et al. Severe Cutaneous Psoriasis after Certolizumab Pegol Treatment: Report of a Case. *Am. J. Gastroenterol.* 2009;104:2867-8.

[50] Klein RQ, Spivack J, Choate KA, et al. Psoriatic Skin Lesions Induced by Certolizumab Pegol. *Arch. Dermatol.* 2010;146:1055-6.

[51] Pirard D, Arco D, Debrouckere V, et al. Anti-tumor necrosis factor alpha-induced psoriasiform eruptions: three further cases and current overview. *Dermatology* 2006;213:182-6.

[52] Gordon KB, Langley RG, Leonardi C, et al. Clinical response to adalimumab treatment in patients with moderate to severe psoriasis: double-blind, randomized controlled trial and open-label extension study. *J. Am. Acad. Dermatol.* 2006;55:598-606.

[53] Menter A, Tyring S, Gordon K, et al. Adalimumab therapy for moderate to severe psoriasis: a randomized, controlled phase III trial. *J. Am. Acad. Dermatol.* 2008;58:106-15.

[54] Mease P, Gladman D, Ritchlin C, et al. Adalimumab for the treatment of patients with moderately to severely active psoriatic arthritis. *Arthritis Rheum.* 2005;52:3279-89.

[55] Gladman D, Mease P, Ritchlin C, et al. Adalimumab for long-term treatment of psoriatic arthritis. Forty-eight week data from the adalimumab effectiveness in psoriatic arthritis trials. *Arthritis Rheum.* 2007;56:476-88.

[56] Gottlieb A, Korman NJ, Gordon KB, et al. Guidelines of care for the management of psoriasis and psoriatic arthritis: Section 2. Psoriatic arthritis: Overview and guidelines of care for treatment with an emphasis on the biologics. *J. Am. Acad. Dermatol.* 2008;58:851-64.

[57] Krueger GG, Langley RG, Finlay AY, et al. Patient-reported outcomes of psoriasis improvement with etanercept therapy: results of a randomized phase III trial. *Br J Dermatol* 2005;153:1192-9.

[58] Moore A, Gordon KB, Kang S, et al. A randomized, open-label trial of continuous versus interrupted etanercept therapy in the treatment of psoriasis. *J. Am. Acad. Dermatol.* 2007;56:598-603.

[59] Leonardi CL, Powers JL, Matheson RT, et al. Etanercept as monotherapy in patients with psoriasis. *N Engl J Med* 2003;349:2014-22.

[60] Mease PJ, Kivitz AJ, Burch FX, et al. Etanercept treatment of psoriatic arthritis: safety, efficacy, and effect on disease progression. *Arthritis Rheum.* 2004;50:2264-72.

[61] Matsuno H, Yudoh K, Katayama R, et al. The role of TNF-alpha in the pathogenesis of inflammation and joint destruction in rheumatoid arthritis (RA): a study using a human RA/ SCID mouse chimera. *Rheumatology (Oxford)* 2002;41:329-37.

[62] Chaudhari U, Romano P, Mulcahy LD, et al. Efficacy and safety of infliximab monotherapy for plaque-type psoriasis: a randomized trial. *Lancet* 2001;357:1842-7.

[63] Gottlieb AB, Evans R, Li S, et al. Infliximab induction therapy for patients with severe plaque-type psoriasis: a randomized, double-blind, placebo-controlled trial. *J. Am. Acad. Dermatol.* 2004;51:534-42.

[64] Reich K, Nestle FO, Papp K, et al. Infliximab induction and maintenance therapy for moderate-to-severe psoriasis: a phase III, multicentre, double-blind trial. *Lancet* 2005;366:1367-74.

[65] Antoni CE, Kavanaugh A, Kirkham B, et al. Sustained benefits of infliximab therapy for dermatologic and articular manifestations of psoriatic arthritis: Results from the infliximab multinational psoriatic arthritis controlled trial (IMPACT). *Arthritis Rheum.* 2005;52:1227-36.

[66] Antoni C, Krueger GG, de Vlam K, et al. Infliximab improves signs and symptoms of psoriatic arthritis: results of the IMPACT 2 trial. *Ann Rheum. Dis.* 2005;64:1150-7.

[67] Vermeire S, Norman M, Van Assche G, et al. Effectiveness of concomitant immunosuppressive therapy in suppressing the formation of antibodies to infliximab in Crohn's disease. *Gut* 2007;56:1226-31.

[68] Lecluse LLA, Piskin G, Mekkes JR, et al. Review and expert opinion on prevention and treatment of infliximab-related infusion reactions. *Br. J. Dermatol.* 2008;159:527-36.

[69] Xu Z, Vu P, Lee H, et al. Population pharmacokinetics of golimumab an anti-tumor necrosis factor-α human monoclonal antibody, in patients with psoriatic arthritis. *J. Clin. Pharmacol.* 2009;49:1056-70.

[70] Kavanaugh A, McInnes I, Mease P, et al. Golimumab, a new human tumor necrosis factor α, administered every four weeks as a subcutaneous injection in psoriatic arthritis: twenty-four-week efficacy and safety results of a randomized, placebo-controlled study. *Arthritis Rheum.* 2009;60:976-86.

[71] Ortonne JP, Sterry W, Tasset C, et al. Safety and efficacy of subcutaneous certolizumab pegol, a new anti-TNF-alpha monoclonal antibody, in patients with moderate-to-severe chronic plaque psoriasis: preliminary results from a double-blind placebo-controlled trial. *J. Am. Acad Dermatol.* 2007;56:AB6. Presented at the 65th Annual Meeting of the American Academy of Dermatology (AAAD), February 2-7, 2007.

[72] Heffernan MP, Leonardi CL. Alefacept for Psoriasis. *Semin. Cutan Med. Surg.* 2010;29:53-5.

[73] Weger W. Current status and new developments in the treatment of psoriasis and psoriatic arthritis with biological agents. *Br. J. Pharmacol.* 2010;160:810-20.

[74] Ellis CN, Krueger GG. Treatment of chronic plaque psoriasis by selective targeting of memory effector T lymphocytes. *N. Engl. J. Med.* 2001;345:248-55

[75] Ortonne JP. Clinical response to alefacept: results of a phase 3 study of intramuscular administration of alefacept in patients with chronic plaque psoriasis. *J. Eur. Acad. Dermatol. Venereol.* 2003;17:12-6.

[76] Krueger GG, Papp KA, Stough DB, et al. A randomized, double-blind, placebo-controlled phase III study evaluating efficacy and tolerability of 2 courses of alefacept in patients with chronic plaque psoriasis. *J. Am. Acad. Dermatol.* 2002;47:821-33.

[77] Mease PJ, Reich K. Alefacept in Psoriatic Arthritis Study group: Alefacept with methotrexate for treatment of psoriatic arthritis: Open-label extension of a randomized, double-blind, placebo-controlled study. *J. Am. Acad Dermatol* 2009;60:402-11.

[78] Rozenblit M, Lebwohl M. New biologics for psoriasis and psoriatic arthritis. *Dermatol. Ther.* 2009;22:56-60.

[79] Leonardi CL, Kimball AB, Papp KA, et al. Efficacy and safety of ustekinumab, a human interleukin-12/23 monoclonal antibody, in patients with psoriasis: 76-week results form a randomized, double blind, placebo-controlled trial (PHOENIX 1). *Lancet* 2008;371:1665-74.

[80] Papp KA, Langley RG, Lebwohl M, et al. Efficacy and safety of ustekinumab, a human interleukin-12.23 monoclonal antibody, in patients with psoriasis: 52-week results form a randomized, double-blind, placebo-controlled trial (PHOENIX 2). *Lancet* 2008;371:1675-84.

[81] Kimball AB, Gordon KB, Langely RG, et a*l.* Safety and efficacy of ABT-874, a fully human interleukin 12/23 monoclonal antibody in the treatment of moderate to severe chronic plaque psoriasis. *Arch. Dermatol.* 2008;144:200-7.

In: Arthritis: Types, Treatment and Prevention   ISBN 978-1-61470-719-6
Editor: Marc N. Pelt   © 2012 Nova Science Publishers, Inc.

Chapter V

Treating Osteoarthritis with Intra-Articular High Molecular Weight Hyaluronic Acid from an Earlier Stage

Misato Hashizume and Masahiko Mihara[*]

Product Research Department, Fuji-Gotemba Research Laboratories,
Chugai Pharmaceutical Co., Ltd., Gotemba, Japan

ABSTRACT

Osteoarthritis (OA), one of the most common joint diseases, is characterized by a slow degradation of cartilage over a long period. OA of the hip and knee causes chronic disability because of the related pain and functional impairment. Currently the most widely used treatment in OA is administration of nonsteroidal anti-inflammatory drugs (NSAIDs) from the early stages of the disease to relieve pain. However, although NSAIDs are useful for pain management, there are reports that they might accelerate progression of the disease. Intra-articular injections of high molecular weight hyaluronic acid (HA) are also used in the treatment of moderate-to-severe OA for pain relief and cartilage protection. HA is a

[*] Corresponding Author: Masahiko Mihara Ph.D. Product Research Department, Chugai Pharmaceutical Co., Ltd., 1-135, Komakado, Gotemba, Shizuoka, 412-8513, Japan. Phone: +81-550-87-6379, Fax: +81-550-87-5397. E-mail: miharamsh@chugai-pharm.co.jp

major component of synovial fluid and plays a central role in joint lubrication; in OA, however, HA levels in the synovial fluid decrease. Several clinical trials have shown that intra-articular HA injections are effective and safe for OA patients who have ongoing pain and who are unable to tolerate other conservative treatments or joint replacement.

We examined the combination effects of intra-articular HA and oral NSAIDs on cartilage degeneration and onset of pain in a rabbit knee OA model. The rabbit OA model was made by partial meniscectomy. A NSAID was administered orally daily for 14 days, starting from the day of meniscectomy. HA was injected intra-articularly into the injured knee every 3 days from the day of surgery. The effect on pain was assessed by an incapacitance tester, and cartilage damage was evaluated by visual assessment and histopathology at 14 days after the surgery. Weight bearing on the injured hind paw decreased time-dependently in the control group. In the HA, NSAID, and HA+NSAID groups, this decrease in hind paw weight bearing was suppressed, demonstrating an analgesic effect. Visible damage and histopathological findings of cartilage degeneration were evident in the cartilages of the control group at day 14. In the HA group, the area of damaged cartilage decreased and cartilage degeneration was ameliorated. In contrast, in the NSAID group, surprisingly, the cartilage degeneration was exacerbated compared with the control group. The exacerbated cartilage degeneration induced by the NSAID was reversed by the concomitant use of HA. The levels of **matrix metalloproteinases (MMP)** -1, MMP-3, and MMP-13 in synovial fluid from the NSAID group were significantly higher than in controls. The increased production of MMPs induced by NSAIDs was counteracted by the concomitant administration of HA.

To analyze the phenomenon of MMP production in the rabbit OA model, we further studied the effects of HA and NSAIDs on the production of **MMPs** from human chondrocytes in vitro. Chondrocytes were cultured with an NSAID and HA in the presence of interleukin (IL)-1β or IL-6+sIL-6R for 24 h. After culture, the production of MMPs, IL-1β, and IL-6 were measured. Our results clearly showed that HA inhibited NSAID-accelerated MMP production, which was followed by production of inflammatory cytokines from cytokine-activated chondrocytes. These results warrant further evaluation of the potential chondroprotective effects of co-administration of HA with NSAIDs.

There are many reports describing the biological activities of HA other than those deriving from its viscoelastic properties. HA has an inhibitory effect on IL-1- or lipopolysaccharide-induced production of inflammatory mediators. Overproduction of IL-6 was observed in OA synovial fluids; therefore, we investigated whether IL-6 induced MMP production. Moreover, we examined whether HA inhibits IL-6-induced MMP production and, if so how HA inhibits IL-6 signaling. Pre-treatment of cells with HA reduced IL-6-induced MMP production and the phosphorylation of extracellular-signal-regulated kinase (ERK). Expression levels of mitogen-activated protein kinase phosphatase (MKP-1), a negative regulator of ERK1/2, was increased in IL-6-treated chondrocytes. Our study was the first to demonstrate that HA suppressed induction of MMPs by IL-6 in human chondrocytes via induction of MKP-1.

Our study and other studies showed that the viscosupplementation and anti-inflammatory effects of HA are clearly involved in improving the symptoms of OA with a very favorable safety profile. Although current guidelines recommend the use of HA only after the unsuccessful use of NSAIDs, we demonstrated that concomitant use of HA is beneficial for reducing the adverse effects of NSAIDs. It is suggested that HA-based therapy from an earlier stage be recommended due to its role in preserving joint functions and maintaining the quality of life of OA patients.

Keywords: high molecular weight hyaluronic acid, analgesic effect, prevention of cartilage degeneration, nonsteroidal anti-inflammatory drugs

INTRODUCTION

Osteoarthritis (OA) is a degenerative joint disease caused by the breakdown and eventual loss of cartilage in one or more joints. OA is the most common form of arthritis and is the most common cause of chronic pain, affecting more than 150 million individuals worldwide. A combination of factors can contribute to osteoarthritis, including being overweight, aging, joint injury or stress, heredity, and muscle weakness. OA commonly affects the hands, spine, hips, and knees. Involvement of OA in the large weight-bearing joints of the hip or knee causes chronic disability because of the related pain and functional impairment.

The most evident morphological sign of OA is the progressive degeneration of articular cartilage, and inflammation may play a role in the progression of cartilage degeneration [1]. Epidemiological studies show a clear link between the progression of tibiofemoral cartilage damage and the presence of a reactive or inflammatory synovium [2, 3]. Over-loading joints produces physiological mechanical stimulation of chondrocytes, resulting in turn in catabolic stimulation by pro-inflammatory cytokines such as interleukin (IL)-1β, tumor necrosis factor-α (TNF-α), and IL-6. Increased numbers of mononuclear cells are observed in synovial tissue, leading to the induction of cytokines and the production of proteases which target the cartilage extracellular matrix [4, 5]. Indeed, the concentrations of IL-1β, TNF-α, and IL-6 in synovial fluid of OA patients are elevated compared with concentrations in healthy subjects [6, 7]. Moreover, expressions of IL-1 receptor I and TNF receptor I are increased in OA chondrocytes and synovial fibroblasts, and the concentration of soluble IL-6 receptor is increased in OA synovial fluid [7-9].

So far, no curative therapeutics (that is, agents that can halt disease progression and reverse any damage) are available for OA. The main goals of current OA therapy are the control of pain and improvement of joint function. Currently available pharmacological therapies for OA mainly target palliation of pain, and these include analgesics, intra-articular therapy, and topical treatments [10]. Nonsteroidal anti-inflammatory drugs (NSAIDs) are widely used for the treatment of OA patients. NSAIDs induce their analgesic and anti-inflammatory effects by suppressing the production of prostaglandins (PGs) via the inhibition of cyclooxygenases (COXs). Although NSAIDs are useful for pain management, there are many reports describing the possibility that they can accelerate progression of the disease [11-14]. Huskisson et al. reported that indomethacin increased the rate of radiological deterioration of joint space in patients with OA of the knee compared with a placebo [11]. In another paper examining 1695 patients in the Rotterdam study, Reijman et al. reported that long-term use of diclofenac might induce accelerated progression of hip and knee OA [14]. In addition, because NSAIDs inhibit COX-1 which regulates platelet activation, gastrointestinal protection, and kidney function, use of NSAIDs increases the incidence of gastrointestinal and renal adverse effects. Moreover two large trials, designed to evaluate adverse effects occurring with NSAIDs in patients with arthritis, reported a higher incidence of myocardial infarction such as heart attack, thrombosis, and stroke due to a relative increase in thromboxane [15, 16]. Given the possibility of cartilage degeneration and the cardiovascular, gastrointestinal, and renal side-effects of NSAIDs, it would be wise to clinically limit their use.

Intra-articular injections of sodium hyaluronate (HA) are used for patients with pain more severe than can be treated with NSAIDs. Several clinical trials have shown that HA therapy is a reasonable treatment for patients with mild-to-moderate OA of the knee and who are suffering from ongoing pain or are unable to tolerate other conservative treatments or a joint replacement operation [17-19]. HA is a major component of the synovial fluid, and increases the viscosity of the fluid. Along with lubricin, it is one of the fluid's main lubricating components. However, HA in the synovial fluids of OA patients is reduced accompanying inflammation. Therefore, the purpose of intra-articular HA therapy is to make up for the loss of viscoelasticity of synovial fluid accompanying inflammation and to protect against the degradation of cartilage. Regarding the viscoelastic properties of HA, it is thought that higher molecular weight HA is superior to lower molecular weight HA [20]. Although the half-life of HA injected into the joints is relatively short at approx. 12 h to approx. 2 days, depending on its molecular mass [21, 22], the clinical benefits are retained for weeks to months and delay OA progression by more than 1 year [23, 24]. Therefore, it is highly possible that HA shows its efficacy in OA therapy via not only its viscoelastic properties but also through other biological activities. Indeed, it is reported that HA suppresses the production of MMPs, which break down articular cartilage from chondrocytes and synovial cells, through binding with CD44 [25].

In this article, we first examine the combined effects of intra-articular HA and NSAIDs on cartilage degeneration and pain using a rabbit OA model, and we then examine the mechanisms underlying the cartilage protective action of HA. We also briefly examine the pharmacological features and the adverse effects of HA of different molecular weights.

ANALGESIC AND CARTILAGE PROTECTIVE EFFECTS OF HA AND NSAIDS

Rabbit OA Model

The experimental rabbit OA model was made by partial meniscectomy in the left hind paw according to the modification of Colombo's method reported by Kikuchi et al. [26]. Loxoprofen monosodium as a NSAID was orally administered daily from the day of meniscectomy for 14 days. The first dose was administered immediately after the surgery. SUVENYL® (High molecular weight 2700kDa HA [SVE]) as a high molecular weight HA was intra-articularly injected 5 times (day 0, 3, 6, 9, 12) at a dose of 0.1 mL/kg to the meniscectomized left cavity of the knee joint. The control group received water orally and intra-articular saline. The NSAID group received the NSAID orally and intra-articular saline. The HA group received water orally and intra-articular SVE. The NSAID+HA group received the NSAID orally and intra-articular SVE.

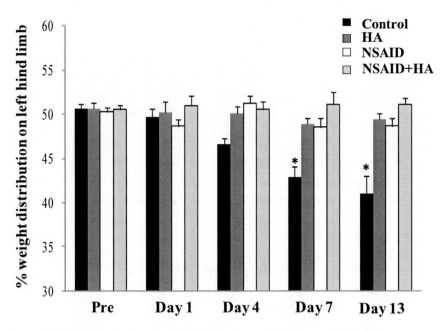

Figure 1. Weight distribution on left hind paw in a rabbit OA model. Weight distribution on left hind paw was measured by Incapacitance Tester 1–2 h after NSAID administration. Columns and error bars indicate the mean and SE of 8 animals. Statistical analysis was by Dunnett's test (*: $p < 0.05$).

Analgesic Effect

Pain was assessed by means of an incapacitance tester (Linton Instrumentation, Norfolk, England) which independently measures the weight bearing on each hind paw. It has been reported that the analgesic effects of morphine and celecoxib could be quantitatively assessed in this system [27], and this method has been utilized for the evaluation of anti-OA drugs and analgesic drugs [28, 29]. The analgesic effect of the NSAID and HA is shown in Figure 1. The control group showed a time dependent decrease in the percentage of weight distribution on the left hind paw—the paw that had been operated on—because of pain.

In contrast, in the other three groups, the values prior to the surgery were generally maintained at all measurement times, demonstrating that both NSAID and HA have an analgesic effect. This analgesic effect was observed when NSAID and HA were administered after onset of pain [30].

It is well-known that PGs play a crucial role in pain and inflammation. Higher levels of PGE_2 are observed in the cartilage of OA patients than in normal cartilage [31].

NSAIDs are potent inhibitors of PG production thereby inducing an analgesic effect. It has been reported that HA also inhibited PGE_2 production in synovial fluid of rheumatoid arthritis (RA) patients [32]. Therefore, inhibition of PGE_2 production might be one of the mechanisms underlying the analgesic effects of HA.

Cartilage Degeneration

Cartilage damage was assessed visually and histopathologically. For visual assessment, the resected left lateral condyle of the femur was covered with plastic wrap, and the area of damage was measured by tracing the area of injury, which consisted of rough white areas of cartilage with a coarse surface and hollow areas with pitted cartilage tissue.

The original tracing was scanned and then analyzed by computer. For histopathological assessment, the **safranin-O** unstained area, which indicates a loss of proteoglycans from the joint cartilage, was measured with a 20× eyepiece micrometer (1 mm reticle divided into 20 units).

In the visual assessment, both the rough white area and the hollow area were significantly higher in the NSAID group than in the control group. The NSAID+HA group had a significantly lower value for both areas than the NSAID group.

The HA group had a lower (but not significantly lower) value for the rough white area and a significantly lower value for the hollow area compared with the control group. In the histopathological assessment the NSAID group had an increased **safranin-O** unstained area compared with the control group, however both the NSAID+HA group and the control group had a greater **safranin-O** unstained area compared with the HA group (Figure 2).

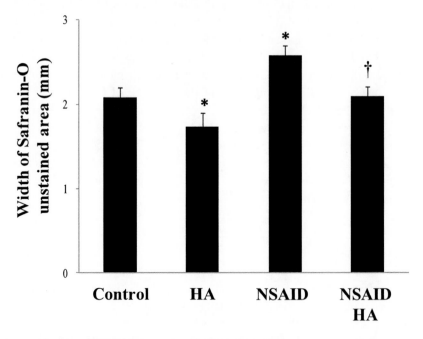

Figure 2. **Safranin-O** unstained area of cartilage in a rabbit OA model. Width of Safranin O unstained area (mm) was measured by using a 20× eyepiece micrometer and counting the divisions on the reticle. Columns and error bars indicate the mean and SE of 8 animals. Statistical analysis was by unpaired t-test. The HA group or the NSAID group was compared with the control group (*: $p < 0.05$). The NSAID+HA group was compared with the NSAID group (†: $p < 0.05$).

EFFECT OF HA AND NSAIDs ON CHONDROCYTES

Kikuchi et al. reported that HA acted to protect cartilage in a rabbit OA model [26]. We confirmed their results in our study. On the other hand, to our surprise, NSAIDs increased the visibly damaged area and exacerbated cartilage degeneration compared with the control group. This supports the clinical findings that NSAIDs accelerate progression of OA [11-14]. Although the precise reasons for this phenomenon are not clear, there are two possible mechanisms: One is that the analgesic effect enables normal movement but, without improvement in the viscoelastic properties of the synovial fluid, this may then lead to increased abrasion at the joint surface. The other is that NSAIDs directly induce cartilage degeneration. There are reports in which NSAIDs are described as inhibiting the matrix biosynthesis of the joint cartilage [11-14].

MMP LEVELS IN SYNOVIAL FLUIDS IN THE RABBIT OA MODEL

To clarify how NSAIDs augmented cartilage degeneration in the rabbit OA model, we measured the levels of MMPs in synovial lavage fluid from OA rabbits in which NSAID treatment had accelerated cartilage destruction (Figure 3). MMPs are proteases that participate in irreparable proteolysis and remodeling of the extracellular matrix, and it is reported that their levels are clearly elevated in OA and RA patients [33, 34]. The levels of MMPs in synovial fluid from the NSAID group were much higher than those from the control group, but this NSAID-induced augmentation of MMP production was suppressed by combination with HA. These facts strongly suggest that elevated production of MMPs might be a cause of the accelerated cartilage destruction observed with NSAID treatment.

MMP PRODUCTION FROM CHONDROCYTES IN VITRO

Next we examined the effect of NSAIDs and HA on MMP production from chondrocytes. Human chondrocytes derived from normal human articular cartilage were cultured for 24 h. After confluence, the cells were stimulated with IL-1β or IL-6+sIL-6R for 24 h in the presence or absence of an NSAID (celecoxib or indomethacin) with or without HA. Culture supernatants were then collected and MMPs, IL-1β, IL-6, and PGE_2 concentrations in the supernatants were measured. It is reported that increased levels of IL-1 are detected in synovial fluids of OA and RA patients [6], and that IL-1 stimulates the mitogen-activated protein kinase (MAPK) family and promotes the expression of MMPs in human chondrocytes [35-37]. IL-6 is also abundant in

OA and RA synovial fluids, and these high levels of IL-6 are associated with an increased risk of cartilage loss (as assessed by MRI) [38]. Moreover, IL-6 induces MMPs from synovial fibroblasts and chondrocytes [39]. Based on these lines of evidence, we used IL-6 as well as IL-1 in our study to stimulate chondrocytes.

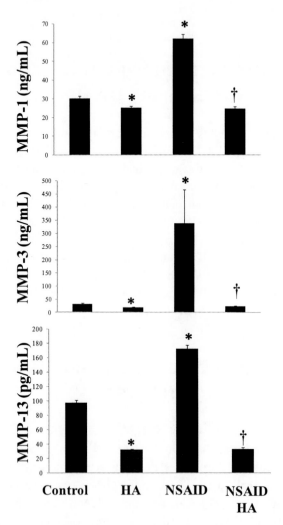

Figure 3. MMP levels in synovial lavage fluid from a rabbit OA model. Synovial lavage fluid was collected and MMPs were measured by ELISA. Columns and error bars indicate the mean and SE of 7 animals. Statistical analysis was by unpaired t-test. The HA group or the NSAID group was compared with the control group (*: $p < 0.05$). The NSAID+HA group was compared with the NSAID group (†: $p < 0.05$).

NSAIDs significantly enhanced the production of MMP-1, MMP-3, and MMP-13 from chondrocytes stimulated with IL-1β or IL-6+sIL-6R, although NSAIDs did not induce their production directly. Furthermore, NSAIDs also augmented IL-1β and IL-6 production from chondrocytes after stimulation with these cytokines. PGE_2 production by IL-1β and IL-6+sIL-6R was completely inhibited by the NSAIDs. There are reports indicated that the suppression of PGE_2 concentration leads to chondroprotective effects [40]. In contrast, PGE_2 is reported to participate in synthesis and degradation of cartilage matrix [41, 42]. PGE_2 is known to bind to four distinct cell surface receptors (EP1, EP2, EP3, and EP4), and it is reported that EP2 and EP4 receptor signaling inhibits the expression of MMP-13 in human chondrocytes induced by IL-1β and TNF-α [43-45]. Therefore, we examined whether PGE_2 counteracts NSAID-induced augmentation of MMP production. However, the addition of PGE_2 did not reverse MMP production, suggesting that the reduction of PGE_2 by NSAIDs is not related to the augmentation of MMP production. The mechanisms behind this phenomenon remain to be investigated in the future. Based on these lines of evidence, the mechanism of cartilage destruction by NSAIDs is suggested to be as follows: (step 1) NSAIDs augment IL-1β and IL-6 production from cytokine-activated chondrocytes; (step 2) IL-1β and IL-6 induce MMP production; and (step 3) the MMPs cause cartilage damage.

HA inhibited cytokine-induced production of MMP-1, MMP-3, and MMP-13, and similar results are reported by others [46-48]. Moreover, HA suppressed NSAID-augmented MMP productions and NSAID-augmented productions of IL-1β and IL-6. These results explain how HA inhibited the augmentation of cartilage destruction by NSAID in the rabbit OA model (Figure 4).

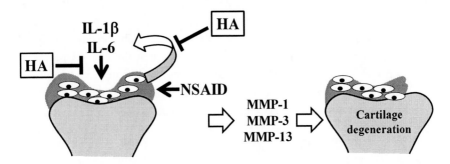

Figure 4. Scheme of the effect of HA on NSAID-augmented MMP production.

THE MECHANISM OF HA SUPPRESSION OF CYTOKINE SIGNALING

HA inhibits IL-1 signaling and suppresses production of inflammatory cytokines and other inflammatory mediators such as MMP-1, MMP-3, and MMP-13 [49]. We also showed that HA inhibited IL-6 signaling to induce MMP-1, MMP-3, MMP-13, and IL-6 production in human chondrocytes.

However, very little is known concerning the mechanism by which HA signaling exerts its biological activity. Recently, Yatabe et al. reported that HA reduced IL-1α-stimulated phosphorylation of IL-1 receptor-associated kinase 1 (IRAK1) and extracellular signal-regulated protein kinase1/2 (ERK1/2) through the induction of IRAK-M, a negative regulator of IRAK1, via CD44 signaling [50]. The induction of IRAK-M by HA caused a reduction of IL-1α-induced ADAMTS4 (aggrecanase-1) production. Another group has reported that HA suppresses IL-1β-enhanced MMP-1 and MMP-3 synthesis in RA synovial fibroblasts via ICAM-1 through down-regulation of NF-κB and p38 [48]. On the other hand, there are no studies to show how HA inhibits IL-6-induced MMP production.

IL-6 signal transduction through gp130 activates members of the Janus kinase family, resulting in the activation of both the signal transducer and activator of transcription (STAT) and MAPK pathways [51, 52]. We therefore investigated whether the STAT or MAPK pathway is involved in IL-6+sIL-6R-induced MMP production using STAT inhibitor and MEK/ERK inhibitor. Stimulation of chondrocytes with IL-6+sIL-6R induced both STAT3 and ERK phosphorylation, and there were clear reductions in the phospho-signals by STAT inhibitor and MEK/ERK inhibitor, respectively.

After pre-incubation with STAT inhibitor or MEK/ERK inhibitor, cells were stimulated with IL-6+sIL-6R for 24 h, and then MMP-1, MMP-3, and MMP-13 concentrations were measured. The MEK/ERK inhibitor blocked MMP production by IL-6+sIL-6R, but the STAT inhibitor only marginally influenced production of these factors, suggesting that the MAPK pathway is dominantly responsible for MMP induction by IL-6. Since STAT inhibitor also inhibits NF-κB as well as STAT, NF-κB inhibition might participate in the slight inhibition of MMP production observed by STAT inhibitor. Consistent with our data, Legendre et al. also reported that MEK/ERK inhibitor as well as STAT inhibitor inhibited IL-6+sIL-6R-induced MMP gene expression [53].

HA Blocks IL-6+sIL-6R-Induced MMP Production via CD44

It has been reported that HA can associate with several cell surface proteins, such as CD44 [54] and ICAM-1 [55], and that each receptor could be involved in the inhibition of MMP production depending on cell stimulants or producer cell types [56, 57]. In fact, it is reported that IL-1-induced MMP production is inhibited by HA and that this inhibitory effect of HA is reversed by anti-CD44 antibody and anti-ICAM-1 antibody [48]. Therefore, we examined whether anti-CD44 antibody or anti-ICAM-1 antibody also reversed HA-induced suppression of MMP induction by IL-6. IL-6+sIL-6R induced a marked increase in MMP production, and HA significantly suppressed this IL-6+sIL-6R-induced MMP production. The inhibitory effect of HA on IL-6+sIL-6R-induced MMP production was decreased by anti-CD44 antibody, but not by anti-ICAM-1 antibody. The reason for this discrepancy between IL-1 and IL-6 is unclear and further study is necessary.

Effect of HA on the IL-6+sIL-6R-Induced Phosphorylation of MEK and ERK

The IL-6+IL-6R complex associates with gp130 leading to initiation of signaling, followed by binding of membrane-associated GTPases with Raf-1 (MAP kinase kinase kinase). After binding, Raf-1 can be phosphorylated to activate the dual-specificity protein kinase MEK1/2 (MAP kinase kinase) which in turn is phosphorylated to activate ERK1/2 (MAP kinase) through sequential protein phosphorylation [58]. Activated ERKs are pleiotropic effectors of cell physiology and control gene expression.

We tested whether HA blocked the phosphorylation of MEK and ERK. We found that IL-6+sIL-6R induced the phosphorylation of both MEK and ERK, but HA inhibited only ERK phosphorylation. This means that in the presence of HA, activation of the MAPK pathway was halted in ERK. Negative regulation of MAPK activity is mediated by MAPK phosphatase, which dephosphorylates MAPK at threonine and tyrosine residues. So we then examined the influence of HA on MKP-1 expression.

We also showed that HA induced MKP-1 expression in **IL-6+sIL-6R-**treated and untreated cells. Furthermore, IL-6+sIL-6R induced MKP-1 protein. To determine the involvement of MKP-1 in HA-induced suppression of MMP production, we tested whether an MKP-1 inhibitor blocked the effect of HA. The MKP-1 inhibitor clearly reversed the suppressive effect of HA on MMP production, to the level of medium control. Moreover, in chondrocytes with MKP-1 knocked-down, production of MMPs was partially inhibited. We obtained the same results for MMP-1, MMP-3, and MMP-13. From these results, it is thought that HA inhibited IL-6+sIL-6R-induced MMP production by up-regulating MKP-1 expression. This idea is strongly supported by the fact that MKP-1 inhibitors and MKP-1 siRNA completely prevented the suppressive effect of HA on the IL-6+sIL-6R-induced MMP production (Figure 5).

The IL-1 signal via the IL-1 receptor I is transduced by IRAK1 and subsequently induces phosphorylation of ERK1/2. Therefore, induction of MKP-1 by HA might be a mechanism of inhibition of IL-1 signaling other than by the induction of IRAK-M and by direct inhibition of NF-κB, as described previously [48, 50].

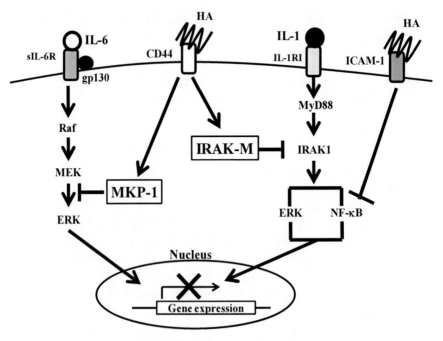

Figure 5. Hypothesized signaling pathways for HA inhibition of cytokine signaling.

PHARMACOLOGICAL FEATURES OF HA

The Pharmacological Effects of HA of Different Molecular Weights

There are several HA products for intra-articular injection currently available all over the world. The molecular weight of HA is different among these products, ranging from 500 kDa to more than 6 million Da. It is well-known that high molecular weight HA is superior to low molecular weight HA in terms of viscoelastic and elastic properties [59]. However, although many pre-clinical studies have shown that high molecular weight HA (2700 kDa) more effectively inhibits the expression of ADAMTS-4, MMP-1, IL-1, and TNF-α than does low molecular weight HA (approx. 800 kDa) [48, 50, 60], there have been no clinical studies to compare the efficacies of HA of different molecular weights. Further studies are necessary to clarify the issue.

The Tolerability of HA

Some HA products, such as Supartz® (Artz®) and Synvisc® are extracted from rooster combs, and a contraindication to treatment would be an allergy to eggs or chicken. On the other hand, SUVENYL® and Euflexxa® are made by fermentative processes and there is no limitation to their use. Local adverse effects such as injection site pain occur with a low incidence on a per-patient or per-injection basis with all types of HA (0–12.8% per patient; 0–2.8% per injection) [61–63]. Local adverse events are typically mild-to-moderate in nature; moreover, they often resolve spontaneously or after treatment of symptoms. Local adverse events do not result in any long-term sequelae [64].

CONCLUSION

Current guidelines for the treatment of knee OA recommend the use of HA only after patients have not responded to non-pharmacologic therapies and simple analgesics, and after the unsuccessful use of nonselective and COX-2 selective NSAIDs. Given the concern about cartilage destruction, as well as side effects associated with the use of NSAIDs, the use of HA earlier in OA treatment should be considered. While no study has been specifically designed to evaluate the earlier use of HA for treating OA, several lines of evidence strongly suggest that HA is more effective when used in the earlier stages of the disease.

A retrospective study by Lussier and colleagues found that patients with a lower grade of OA showed a better or much better overall response to HA therapy than did patients with a higher grade of OA [65]. Another retrospective study showed that pooled visual analog scale scores for patients with grade III OA were significantly better than those for patients with grade IV OA when patients were treated with HA [66]. Finally, in a study of 4253 patients with knee OA, the benefit of early HA therapy was apparent: HA therapy seemed to be more effective in patients who were more recently diagnosed (within 1 year) compared with those who had more time since diagnosis [67]. Collectively, these studies support the idea that the use of HA from an earlier stage in the OA treatment paradigm, shortly after diagnosis of OA, be strongly recommended.

From our own studies and other studies it is clear that HA, through its viscosupplementation and anti-inflammatory effects, is involved in the improvement of symptoms of OA and has a very favorable safety profile. Although current guidelines recommend the use of HA only after the unsuccessful use of NSAIDs, we showed that concomitant use of HA is beneficial for reducing the adverse effects of NSAIDs. It is suggested that HA therapy from an earlier stage be recommended due to its role in preserving joint functions and maintaining the quality of life of OA patients.

REFERENCES

[1]   Benito MH, Veale DJ, FitzGerald O, van den Berg WB, Bresnihan B. Synovial tissue inflammation in early and late osteoarthritis. *Ann. Rheum. Dis.* 2005;64:1263–7.

[2]   Ayral X, Pickering EH, Woodworth TG, Mackillop N, Dougados M. Synovitis: a potential predictive factor of structural progression of medial tibiofemoral knee osteoarthritis — results of a 1 year longitudinal arthroscopic study in 422 patients. *Osteoarthritis Cartilage.* 2005;13:361–7.

[3]   Pozgan U, Caglic D, Rozman B, Nagase H, Turk V, Turk B. Expression and activity profiling of selected cysteine cathepsins and matrix

metalloproteinases in synovial fluids from patients with rheumatoid arthritis and osteoarthritis. *Biol. Chem.* 2010;391:571–9.

[4]   Rollín R, Marco F, Jover JA, García-Asenjo JA, Rodríguez L, López-Durán L, Fernández-Gutiérrez B. Early lymphocyte activation in the synovial microenvironment in patients with osteoarthritis: comparison with rheumatoid arthritis patients and healthy controls. *Rheumatol. Int.* 2008;28:757–64.

[5]   Da RR, Qin Y, Baeten D, Zhang Y. B cell clonal expansion and somatic hypermutation of Ig variable heavy chain genes in the synovial membrane of patients with osteoarthritis. *J. Immunol.* 2007;178:557–65.

[6]   Martel-Pelletier, J., Lajeunesse, D., Pelletier, J.P. In: Arthritis and Allied Conditions. *A Textbook of Rheumatology 15th edn.* 2005; pp. 2199–2226.

[7]   Kaneko S, Satoh T, Chiba J, Ju C, Inoue K, Kagawa J. Interleukin-6 and interleukin-8 levels in serum and synovial fluid of patients with osteoarthritis. *Cytokines Cell Mol. Ther.* 2000;6:71–9.

[8]   Sadouk MB, Pelletier JP, Tardif G, Kiansa K, Cloutier JM, Martel-Pelletier J. Human synovial fibroblasts coexpress IL-1 receptor type I and type II mRNA. The increased level of the IL-1 receptor in osteoarthritic cells is related to an increased level of the type I receptor. *Lab. Invest.* 1995;73:347–55.

[9]   Alaaeddine N, DiBattista JA, Pelletier JP, Cloutier JM, Kiansa K, Dupuis M, Martel-Pelletier J. Osteoarthritic synovial fibroblasts possess an increased level of tumor necrosis factor-receptor 55 (TNF-R55) that mediates biological activation by TNF-alpha. *J. Rheumatol.* 1997;24:1985–94.

[10] American College of Rheumatology Subcommittee on Osteoarthritis Guidelines. Recommendations for the medical management of osteoarthritis of the hip and knee. *Arthritis Rheum: 2000 update,* 2000;43:1905–15.

[11] Huskisson EC, Berry H, Gishen P, Jubb RW, Whitehead J. Effects of antiinflammatory drugs on the progression of osteoarthritis of the knee. LINK Study Group. Longitudinal Investigation of Nonsteroidal Antiinflammatory Drugs in Knee Osteoarthritis. *J. Rheumatol.* 1995;22:1941–6.

[12] Rashad S, Revell P, Hemingway A, Low F, Rainsford K, Walker F. Effect of non-steroidal anti-inflammatory drugs on the course of osteoarthritis. *Lancet.* 1989;2:519–22.

[13] Dougados M, Gueguen A, Nguyen M, Berdah L, Lequesne M, Mazieres B, Vignon E. Radiological progression of hip osteoarthritis: definition, risk factors and correlations with clinical status. *Ann. Rheum. Dis.* 1996;55:356–62.

[14] Reijman M, Bierma-Zeinstra SM, Pols HA, Koes BW, Stricker BH, Hazes JM. Is there an association between the use of different types of nonsteroidal antiinflammatory drugs and radiologic progression of osteoarthritis? The Rotterdam Study. *Arthritis Rheum.* 2005;52:3137–42.

[15] Bombardier C, Laine L, Reicin A, Shapiro D, Burgos-Vargas R, Davis B, Day R, Ferraz MB, Hawkey CJ, Hochberg MC, Kvien TK, Schnitzer TJ; VIGOR Study Group. Comparison of upper gastrointestinal toxicity of rofecoxib and naproxen in patients with rheumatoid arthritis. VIGOR Study Group. *N. Engl. J. Med.* 2000;343:1520–8.

[16] Bird HA, Clarke AK, Fowler PD, Little S, Podgorski MR, Steiner J. An assessment of tenoxicam, a nonsteroidal anti-inflammatory drug of long half-life, in patients with impaired renal function suffering from osteoarthritis or rheumatoid arthritis. *Clin. Rheumatol.* 1989;8:453–60.

[17] Petrella RJ, DiSilvestro MD, Hildebrand C. Effects of hyaluronate sodium on pain and physical functioning in osteoarthritis of the knee. A randomized, double-blind, placebo-controlled clinical trial. *Arch. Intern Med.* 2002;162:292–8.

[18] Dougados M, Nguyen M, Listrat V, Amor B. High molecular weight sodium hyaluronate (hyalectin) in osteoarthritis of the knee: a 1 year placebo-controlled trial. *Osteoarthritis Cartilage.* 1993;1:97–103.

[19] Salk RS, Chang TJ, D'Costa WF, Soomekh DJ, Grogan KA. Sodium hyaluronate in the treatment of osteoarthritis of the ankle: a controlled, randomized, double-blind pilot study. *J. Bone Joint Surg. Am.* 2006;88:295–302.

[20] Kobayashi Y, Okamoto A, Nishinari K. Viscoelasticity of hyaluronic acid with different molecular weights. *Biorheology.* 1994;31:235–44.

[21] Brown TJ, Laurent UB, Fraser JR. Turnover of hyaluronan in synovial joints: elimination of labelled hyaluronan from the knee joint of the rabbit. *Exp. Physiol.* 1991;76:125–34.

[22] Fraser JR, Laurent TC, Laurent UB. Hyaluronan: its nature, distribution, functions and turnover. *J. Intern. Med.* 1997;242:27–33.

[23] Wang CT, Lin J, Chang CJ, Lin YT, Hou SM. Therapeutic effects of hyaluronic acid on osteoarthritis of the knee. A meta-analysis of randomized controlled trials. *J. Bone Joint Surg. Am.* 2004;86-A:538–45.

[24] Listrat V, Ayral X, Patarnello F, Bonvarlet JP, Simonnet J, Amor B, Dougados M. Arthroscopic evaluation of potential structure modifying activity of hyaluronan (Hyalgan) in osteoarthritis of the knee. *Osteoarthritis Cartilage.* 1997;5:153–60.

[25] Wang CT, Lin YT, Chiang BL, Lin YH, Hou SM. High molecular weight hyaluronic acid down-regulates the gene expression of osteoarthritis-associated cytokines and enzymes in fibroblast-like synoviocytes from patients with early osteoarthritis. *Osteoarthritis Cartilage.* 2006;14:1237–47.

[26] Kikuchi T, Yamada H, Shinmei M. Effect of high molecular weight hyaluronan on cartilage degeneration in a rabbit model of osteoarthritis. *Osteoarthritis Cartilage.* 1996;4:99–110.

[27] Pomonis JD, Boulet JM, Gottshall SL, Phillips S, Sellers R, Bunton T, Walker K. Development and pharmacological characterization of a rat model of osteoarthritis pain. *Pain* 2005;114:339–46.

[28] McDougall JJ, Watkins L, Li Z. Vasoactive intestinal peptide (VIP) is a modulator of joint pain in a rat model of osteoarthritis. *Pain* 2006;123:98–105.

[29] Bley KR, Bhattacharya A, Daniels DV, Gever J, Jahangir A, O'Yang C, Smith S, Srinivasan D, Ford AP, Jett MF. RO1138452 and RO3244794: characterization of structurally distinct, potent and selective IP (prostacyclin) receptor antagonists. *Br. J. Pharmacol.* 2006:147;335–45.

[30] Hashizume M, Koike N, Yoshida H, Suzuki M, Mihara M. High molecular weight hyaluronic acid relieved joint pain and prevented the progression of cartilage degeneration in a rabbit osteoarthritis model after onset of arthritis. *Mod. Rheumatol.* 2010;20:432–8.

[31] Jacques C, Sautet A, Moldovan M, Thomas B, Humbert L, Berenbaum F. Cyclooxygenase activity in chondrocytes from osteoarthritic and healthy cartilage. *Rev. Rhum. Engl. Ed.* 1999;66:701–4.

[32] Goto M, Hanyu T, Yoshio T, Matsuno H, Shimizu M, Murata N, Shiozawa S, Matsubara T, Yamana S, Matsuda T. Intra-articular injection of hyaluronate (SI-6601D) improves joint pain and synovial fluid prostaglandin E2 levels in rheumatoid arthritis: a multicenter clinical trial. *Clin. Exp. Rheumatol.* 2001;19:377–83.

[33] Fiedorczyk M, Klimiuk PA, Sierakowski S, Gindzienska-Sieskiewicz E, Chwiecko J. Serum matrix metalloproteinases and tissue inhibitors of metalloproteinases in patients with early rheumatoid arthritis. *J. Rheumatol.* 2006;33:1523–9.

[34] Burrage PS, Mix KS, Brinckerhoff CE. Matrix metalloproteinases: role in arthritis. *Front Biosci.* 2006;11:529–43.

[35] Mengshol JA, Vincenti MP, Coon CI, Barchowsky A, Brinckerhoff CE. Interleukin-1 induction of collagenase 3 (matrix metalloproteinase 13) gene expression in chondrocytes requires p38, c-Jun N-terminal kinase, and nuclear factor kappaB: differential regulation of collagenase 1 and collagenase 3. *Arthritis Rheum.* 2000;43:801–11.

[36] Lefebvre V, Peeters-Joris C, Vaes G. Production of gelatin-degrading matrix metalloproteinases ('type IV collagenases') and inhibitors by articular chondrocytes during their dedifferentiation by serial subcultures and under stimulation by interleukin-1 and tumor necrosis factor alpha. *Biochim. Biophys. Acta.* 1991;1094:8–18.

[37] Reboul P, Pelletier JP, Tardif G, Cloutier JM, Martel-Pelletier J. The new collagenase, collagenase-3, is expressed and synthesized by human chondrocytes but not by synoviocytes. A role in osteoarthritis. *J. Clin. Invest.* 1996;97:2011–9.

[38] Pelletier JP, Raynauld JP, Caron J, Mineau F, Abram F, Dorais M, Haraoui B, Choquette D, Martel-Pelletier J. Decrease in serum level of matrix metalloproteinases is predictive of the disease-modifying effect of osteoarthritis drugs assessed by quantitative MRI in patients with knee osteoarthritis. *Ann. Rheum. Dis.* 2010;69:2095–101.

[39] Jikko A, Wakisaka T, Iwamoto M, Hiranuma H, Kato Y, Maeda T, Fujishita M, Fuchihata H. Effects of interleukin-6 on proliferation and proteoglycan metabolism in articular chondrocyte cultures. *Cell Biol. Int.* 1998;22:615–21.

[40] Nah SS, Choi IY, Lee CK, Oh JS, Kim YG, Moon HB, Yoo B. Effects of advanced glycation end products on the expression of COX-2, PGE2 and NO in human osteoarthritic chondrocytes. *Rheumatology* (Oxford). 2008;47:425–31.

[41] Amin AR, Dave M, Attur M, Abramson SB. COX-2, NO, and cartilage damage and repair. *Curr. Rheumatol. Rep.* 2000;2:447–53.

[42] Goldring MB, Berenbaum F. The regulation of chondrocyte function by proinflammatory mediators: prostaglandins and nitric oxide. *Clin. Orthop. Relat. Res.* 2004;(427 Suppl):S37–46.

[43] Fushimi K, Nakashima S, You F, Takigawa M, Shimizu K. Prostaglandin E2 downregulates TNF-alpha-induced production of matrix metalloproteinase-1 in HCS-2/8 chondrocytes by inhibiting Raf-1/MEK/ERK cascade through EP4 prostanoid receptor activation. *J. Cell Biochem.* 2007;100:783–93.

[44] Sato T, Konomi K, Fujii R, Aono H, Aratani S, Yagishita N, Araya N, Yudoh K, Beppu M, Yamano Y, Nishioka K, Nakajima T. Prostaglandin EP2 receptor signalling inhibits the expression of matrix metalloproteinase 13 in human osteoarthritic chondrocytes. *Ann. Rheum. Dis.* 2011;70:221–6.

[45] Attur M, Al-Mussawir HE, Patel J, Kitay A, Dave M, Palmer G, Pillinger MH, Abramson SB. Prostaglandin E2 exerts catabolic effects in osteoarthritis cartilage: evidence for signaling via the EP4 receptor. *J. Immunol.* 2008;181:5082–8.

[46] Julovi SM, Yasuda T, Shimizu M, Hiramitsu T, Nakamura T. Inhibition of interleukin-1β-stimulated production of matrix metalloproteinases by hyaluronan via CD44 in human articular cartilage. *Arthritis Rheum.* 2004;50:516–25.

[47] Fan Z, Yang H, Bau B, Soder S, Aigner T. Role of mitogen-activated protein kinases and NFκB on IL-1β-induced effects on collagen type II, MMP-1 and 13 mRNA expression in normal articular human chondrocytes. *Rheumatol Int.* 2006;26:900–3.

[48] Yasuda T. Hyaluronan inhibits cytokine production by lipopolysaccharide-stimulated U937 macrophages through down-regulation of NF-κB via ICAM-1. *Inflamm Res.* 2007;56:246–53.

[49] del Fresno C, Otero K, Gómez-García L, González-León MC, Soler-Ranger L, Fuentes-Prior P, Escoll P, Baos R, Caveda L, García F, Arnalich F, López-Collazo E. Tumor cells deactivate human monocytes by up-regulating IL-1 receptor associated kinase-M expression via CD44 and TLR4. *J. Immunol.* 2005;174:3032–40.

[50] Yatabe T, Mochizuki S, Takizawa M, Chijiiwa M, Okada A, Kimura T, Fujita Y, Matsumoto H, Toyama Y, Okada Y. Hyaluronan inhibits expression of ADAMTS4 (aggrecanase-1) in human osteoarthritic chondrocytes. *Ann. Rheum. Dis.* 2009;68:1051–8.

[51] Heinrich PC, Behrmann I, Müller-Newen G, Schaper F, Graeve L. Interleukin-6-type cytokine signalling through the gp130/Jak/STAT pathway. *Biochem. J.* 1998;334: 297–314.

[52] Heinrich PC, Behrmann I, Haan S, Hermanns HM, Müller-Newen G, Schaper F. Principles of interleukin (IL)-6-type cytokine signalling and its regulation. *Biochem. J.* 2003;374:1–20.

[53] Legendre F, Bogdanowicz P, Boumediene K and Pujol JP. Role of interleukin 6 (IL-6)/IL-6R-induced signal tranducers and activators of transcription and mitogen-activated protein kinase/extracellular signal-related kinase in upregulation of matrix metalloproteinase and

ADAMTS gene expression in articular chondrocytes. *J. Rheumatol* 2005;32:1307–16.

[54] Aruffo A, Stamenkovic I, Melnick M, Underhill CB, Seed B. CD44 is the principal cell surface receptor for hyaluronate. *Cell.* 1990;61:303–13.

[55] McCourt PA, Ek B, Forsberg N, Gustafson S. Intercellular adhesion molecule-1 is a cell surface receptor for hyaluronan. *J. Biol. Chem.* 1994;269:30081–4.

[56] Shimizu M, Yasuda T, Nakagawa T, Yamashita E, Julovi SM, Hiramitsu T, Nakamura T. Hyaluronan inhibits matrix metalloproteinase-1 production by rheumatoid synovial fibroblasts stimulated by proinflammatory cytokines. *J. Rheumatol.* 2003;30:1164–72.

[57] Hiramitsu T, Yasuda T, Ito H, Shimizu M, Julovi SM, Kakinuma T, Akiyoshi M, Yoshida M, Nakamura T. Intercellular adhesion molecule-1 mediates the inhibitory effects of hyaluronan on interleukin-1beta-induced matrix metalloproteinase production in rheumatoid synovial fibroblasts via down-regulation of NF-kappaB and p38. *Rheumatology* (Oxford). 2006;45:824–32.

[58] Dong C, Davis RJ, Flavell RA. MAP kinases in the immune response. *Annu. Rev. Immunol.* 2002;20:55–72.

[59] Kato Y, Nakamura S, Nishimura M. Beneficial actions of hyaluronan (HA) on arthritic joints: effects of molecular weight of HA on elasticity of cartilage matrix. *Biorheology.* 2006;43:347–54.

[60] Tanaka M, Masuko-Hongo K, Kato T, Nishioka K, Nakamura H. Suppressive effects of hyaluronan on MMP-1 and RANTES production from chondrocytes. *Rheumatol. Int.* 2006;26:185–90.

[61] Altman RD, Moskowitz R. Intraarticular sodium hyaluronate (Hyalgan) in the treatment of patients with osteoarthritis of the knee: a randomized clinical trial. Hyalgan Study Group. *J. Rheumatol.* 1998;25:2203–12.

[62] Grecomoro G, Martorana U, Di Marco C. Intra-articular treatment with sodium hyaluronate in gonarthrosis: a controlled clinical trial versus placebo. *Pharmatherapeutica.* 1987;5:137–41.

[63] Brzusek D, Petron D. Treating knee osteoarthritis with intra-articular hyaluronans. *Curr. Med. Res. Opin.* 2008;24:3307–22.

[64] Waddell DD. The tolerability of viscosupplementation: low incidence and clinical management of local adverse events. *Curr. Med. Res. Opin.* 2003;19:575–80.

[65] Lussier A, Cividino AA, McFarlane CA, Olszynski WP, Potashner WJ, De Médicis R. Viscosupplementation with hylan for the treatment of osteoarthritis: findings from clinical practice in Canada. *J. Rheumatol.* 1996;23:1579–85.

[66] Waddell DD, Bricker DC. Clinical experience of hylan G-F 20 efficacy in patients with knee osteoarthritis from a large, orthopedic practice. *Arch. Phys Med. Rehabil.* 2003;84:E19.

[67] Kemper F, Gebhardt U, Meng T, Murray C. Tolerability and short-term effectiveness of hylan G-F 20 in 4253 patients with osteoarthritis of the knee in clinical practice. *Curr. Med. Res. Opin.* 2005;21:1261–9.

In: Arthritis: Types, Treatment and Prevention   ISBN 978-1-61470-719-6
Editor: Marc N. Pelt   © 2012 Nova Science Publishers, Inc.

Chapter VI

Subclinical Atherosclerosis in Patients with Rheumatoid and Psoriatic Arthritis

Elisabetta Profumo[*], Brigitta Buttari[*],
Maria Elena Tosti[**], Rossana Scrivo[†], Antonio Spadaro[†],
Chiara Tesori[‡], Manuela Di Franco[†] and Rachele Riganò[*]
[*]Department of Infectious, Parasitic and Immune-mediated Diseases
[**]National Centre of Epidemiology, Surveillance and Health Promotion,
Istituto Superiore di Sanità, Rome
[†] Rheumatology Unit
[‡] Department of Surgical Sciences, University Sapienza,
Rome, Italy

ABSTRACT

Accelerated development of atherosclerosis has been observed in patients with rheumatic diseases such as rheumatoid arthritis (RA) and psoriatic arthritis (PsA). It may be related to the inflammatory overload accompanied to the combination of an excessive production of reactive oxygen species with an impaired antioxidant defence capacity, leading to oxidative stress that may facilitate the development and progression of atherosclerosis. Compared with the general population, patients with RA die prematurely, mainly because of cardiovascular diseases but the mechanism by which premature atherosclerosis develops in RA is unknown. Recent data have demonstrated the prevalence of atherosclerosis also in patients with PsA, a chronic inflammatory autoimmune disease characterized by inflammatory arthritis and skin psoriasis. PsA shares some phenotypic characteristics with RA, even though the synovial inflammation of PsA is characterized by less macrophage infiltration and increased vascularity in comparison to RA inflammation. The increased cardiovascular risk in PsA and RA suggests the need to treat the inflammatory process and to monitor traditional atherosclerotic risk factors in these pathologies.

The aim of our study was to evaluate whether increased oxidative stress may be associated to the presence of subclinical atherosclerosis in patients with RA and in patients with PsA. For this purpose we determined the levels of oxidized low density lipoproteins (ox-LDL) and of nitric oxide (NO) in the sera obtained from 19 patients with RA, 20 with PsA and 20 sex- and age-matched healthy controls. Patients with RA fulfilled the American College of Rheumatology criteria, and patients with PsA fulfilled the CASPAR criteria. In all patients we evaluated the activity and duration of the disease and classical risk factors for atherosclerosis. Our results showed higher levels of ox-LDL and lower levels of NO in sera from patients with RA and PsA than in sera from healthy controls. Notably, higher serum levels of ox-LDL were observed in patients with an intima-media thickness (IMT) >1 than in those with an IMT $\leq$1, and higher serum levels of NO in patients with an IMT $\leq$1 than in those with an IMT >1, in patients with RA and PsA. Our data suggest that monitoring circulating levels of ox-LDL and NO in patients with RA and PsA could give information on the development of atherosclerotic disease and therefore could be useful to the clinical management of patients.

INTRODUCTION

Rheumatoid arthritis (RA) and psoriatic arthritis (PsA) are chronic inflammatory diseases of the musculoskeletal system. In RA the inflammatory process affects the synovium and leads to joint damage and bone destruction [1]. This pathology is characterised by significant morbidity as a result of synovial inflammation and associated disability [2]; it is more frequent in women than in men with a ratio 3:1. The tissue damage is primarily caused by immune complexes and by cell-mediated immunity. In patients affected by RA the synovial joints are characterized by an inflammatory infiltrate, mainly composed by T lymphocytes and monocytes that secrete soluble factors and promote Th1 inflammation, responsible for the tissue damage. Many studies have reported an excess of cardiovascular morbidity and mortality among patients with RA [2]. Compared with the general population, patients with RA die prematurely, mainly because of cardiovascular diseases. In patients with active disease, the majority of cardiovascular deaths are caused by accelerated atherosclerosis [3-6]. Atherosclerosis is a chronic inflammatory disease caused by endothelial dysfunction and characterized by complex interactions between immune and vascular cells. The activation of endothelial cells induces the expression of adhesion molecules on these cells and the recruitment of leucocytes, thus promoting the inflammatory response. Accelerated atherosclerosis observed in patients with RA is probably due to the chronic activation of inflammatory mechanisms involved in this pathology.

Psoriatic arthritis (PsA) is an inflammatory joint disease with heterogeneous presentation and clinical course [7]. Clear evidence exists that this disease is distinct from rheumatoid arthritis and other spondyloarthropathies, based on informations derived from characteristic clinical features, and on data from histopathologic analyses, immunogenetic associations and musculoskeletal imaging. It is usually seronegative for rheumatoid factor. PsA shares some phenotypic characteristics with RA, even though the synovial inflammation of PsA is characterized by less macrophage infiltration and increased vascularity in comparison to RA inflammation. Much interest has been focused previously on the prominent role of T lymphocytes in the inflammatory process; however, many studies strongly support a major contribution of macrophages in the initiation and perpetuation of joint and skin inflammation [7]. Recent data have demonstrated the occurrence of endothelial dysfunction and the prevalence of atherosclerosis also in patients with PsA [8,9]. The occurrence of cardiovascular disease might be directly linked to the cutaneous and musculoskeletal manifestations of this disease involving subsets of circulating monocytes and tissue macrophages activated by inflammatory mediators in the skin and joint [7].

As patients with autoimmune rheumatic diseases live longer due to improved therapies and preventive measures, mortality and disability due to cardiovascular diseases are increasing [10]. The relative risk to develop atherosclerosis is approximately 1.6 in PsA and 3.0 in RA. Increased risks are found when analyzed by atherosclerotic events, causes of death, or surrogate measures of atherosclerosis, such as carotid artery plaque, intima-media thickness (IMT), or coronary artery calcification. As RA and probably PsA predispose to atherosclerosis, an important issue is how to prevent this outcome. Therefore, when considering preventive interventions, the most important question is whether patients with some particular clinical features have greater risk for atherosclerosis. This may suggest that detecting a particular clinical marker will identify patients at high risk for clinical atherosclerosis and may help in establishing a risk prediction model. In the last decade great attention has been focused on the identification of risk factors predisposing to atherosclerotic diseases [11,12]. Many studies have demonstrated correlations of atherosclerosis with clinical conditions characterized by alteration in the metabolism such as diabetes [13] and hypercholesterolemia [14]. Gender is also a risk factor for cardiovascular diseases, as men have higher risk to develop atherosclerosis than women [15], and increasing age is associated with either clinical atherosclerotic events or surrogate markers for atherosclerosis, such as the occurrence of carotid plaque. Of particular interest are the well known associations of the standard measures of acute systemic inflammation such as erythrocyte sedimentation rate (ESR) [16], with atherosclerosis. Evidence exists suggesting that C-reactive protein (CRP) is a particularly consistent predictor of increased risk for atherosclerotic disease in the general population [17]. Traditional risk factors for atherosclerosis are operational in patients with autoimmune rheumatic diseases. Increased incidence of factors such as metabolic syndrome, diabetes and hypertension has been demonstrated in these patients. Furthermore, there may be genetic and environmental risk factors that predispose an individual both to autoimmune disease and to atherosclerosis. It is probably useful to consider certain autoimmune diseases, such as RA, to be equivalent to diabetes in increasing risk for developing atherosclerosis. Of note, among patients with autoimmune diseases, the interpretation of classical risk factors as CRP can be confounded by the correlation with the systemic inflammation that occurs in these pathologies. However, several studies have identified ESR as an independent risk factor for atherosclerosis in patients with RA.

Recently, accumulating evidence has demonstrated the presence of oxidative stress in patients with rheumatic diseases and suggested a role for the use of antioxidants in prevention and treatment of these pathologies [18,19]. It is well known that the inflammatory overload accompanied to the combination of an excessive production of reactive oxygen species with an impaired antioxidant defence capacity, leading to oxidative stress may facilitate the development and progression of atherosclerosis. Furthermore pharmacological control of oxidative stress and stimulation of nitric oxide release have proved to exert beneficial effects also on vascular remodeling in experimental diabetic models [20]. In several vascular disorders, an increase in superoxide (O_2^-) has been shown to contribute to reduced NO bioavailability through its reaction with NO to form peroxynitrite [21].

Thus, it is clear that the cellular redox state is dysregulated, and the resultant generation of reactive oxygen species (ROS) may play important role in driving and possibly initiating the rheumatic disease as well as cardiovascular complications. However, the precise mechanisms of ROS metabolism, and their function in the progression of these pathologies remain largely elusive. The increased cardiovascular risk in PsA and RA suggests the need to treat the inflammatory process and to monitor traditional atherosclerotic risk factors in these pathologies.

Seeking more information on biomarkers for atherosclerosis development in patients with RA and PsA, in our in vitro study we evaluated the possible association of oxidative stress markers in peripheral blood with the presence of subclinical atherosclerosis. For this purpose, we determined by immune enzymatic assays serum levels of oxidized low density lipoproteins (ox-LDL) and NO in patients with RA and PsA divided into two groups according to the presence of atherosclerotic disease determined by echo-color Doppler ultrasonography. As controls we used healthy subjects free of atherosclerotic disease. We also investigated whether these two serum biomarkers were correlated to traditional risk factors for atherosclerosis or to clinical features of the two autoimmune diseases.

MATERIALS AND METHODS

Study Population

We enrolled 19 consecutive patients with RA fulfilling the American College of Rheumatology (ACR) criteria [22] and 20 consecutive patients with PsA fulfilling the Classification Criteria for Psoriatic Arthritis (CASPAR) [23]. We also enrolled 20 sex- and age-matched healthy subjects as controls. Exclusion criteria for patients and controls were recent infection (< 1 month), other autoimmune diseases, malignancy and inflammatory diseases. In all patients we evaluated the activity and duration of the disease and classical risk factors for atherosclerosis (Table). None of the patients and healthy subjects had a history of cardiovascular manifestations. All patients were treated with disease-modifying antirheumatic drugs. Serum samples were obtained from patients and controls and stored at -80°C until use. Informed consent was obtained from all participants.

Table. Baseline characteristics of the 19 patients with rheumatoid arthritis (RA) and of the 20 patients with psoriatic arthritis (PsA)

	Patients with RA	Patients with PsA	P[c]
N	19	20	
Age (years), median (range)	54 (30-64)	51 (35-69)	0.896
Male/female (n)	1/18	13/7	*<0.001*
Duration of the disease (years), median (range)	3 (0.5-25)	7 (1-24)	0.241
Smoking[a], n (%)	7 (37)	5 (25)	0.414
Hypertension[b], n (%)	4 (21)	2 (10)	0.374
Total cholesterol (mg/dl), median (range)	212.5 (160-257)	221 (153-296)	0.409
HDL cholesterol (mg/dl), median (range)	56.5 (45-74)	52 (30-76)	*0.028*
Triglycerids (mg/dl), median (range)	104.5 (90-166)	125 (93-566)	*0.018*
ESR, median (range)	18 (6-40)	10 (3-41)	*0.016*
CRP, median (range)	1.95 (0-43)	0 (0-16)	0.165
IMT >1, n (%)	9 (47)	11 (55)	0.271

[a] Smoking is defined as current smokers;
[b] Hypertension is defined as systolic blood pressure ≥140 mmHg, diastolic blood pressure ≥ 90 mm Hg, or need for hypertensive medication;
[c] Pearson's chi-squared test or Fisher exact test for discrete variables and Mann-Whitney test for continuous variables to evaluate the presence of a statistical significance among patients with RA and PsA;
ESR: erythrocyte sedimentation rate; CRP: C reactive protein; IMT: intima-media thickness.

IMT of the Common Carotid Arteries

To evaluate the presence of atherosclerosis in patients and healthy subjects, IMT of the common carotid arteries was evaluated by Echo-color Doppler. Images were acquired on an ultrasound system equipped with a 7.5 MHz frequency linear-array transducer. The radiologist of the current study was blinded to RA and PsA patients and to the control group, and measurement of the IMT was always performed at the same arterial wall 1 cm proximal to the carotid bifurcation. Two parallel echogenic lines corresponding to the lumen/intima and media/adventitia interfaces were obtained. The distance between these 2 parallel lines corresponded to the IMT. Values were expressed in millimeters.

Serum Ox-LDL and NO Levels

Ox-LDL and NO concentrations in serum samples from patients and healthy subjects were quantified with commercially available ELISA kits (Oxidized LDL Competitive ELISA, Mercodia, Uppsala, Sweden for ox-LDL; Nitrate/Nitrite Colorimetric Assay Kit, Cayman, Lausen Switzerland for NO), as recommended by the manufacturer. The detection limit of the assays were $\leq$ 0.3 U/L for ox-LDL, < 2.5 μM for NO.

Statistical Analysis

Data on serum ox-LDL and NO levels are expressed as medians and inter-quartile ranges. Mann-Whitney non parametric test was used to investigate the significance of unpaired continuous data. Pearson's chi-squared test or Fisher's exact test, when necessary, was used to evaluate the differences in discrete baseline characteristics between groups of patients. Correlations were explored by Spearman rank correlation coefficient. P values less than 0.05 were considered statistically significant.

All the statistical procedures were performed by STATA 8.1 statistical package.

RESULTS

Serum Ox-LDL Levels in RA and PsA Patients

Patients with RA and PsA showed higher ox-LDL concentrations in serum compared to healthy subjects (Figure 1). No differences were observed between patients with RA and PsA in the ox-LDL mean level.

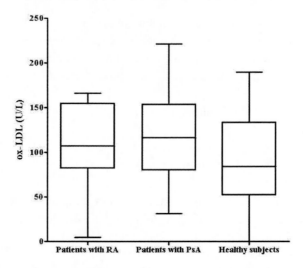

Figure 1. Box plot graphs showing oxidized LDL (ox-LDL) concentrations in serum samples from the 19 patients with rheumatoid arthritis (RA), the 20 patients with psoriatic arthritis (PsA) and the 20 healthy subjects. Patients with RA and PsA showed higher ox-LDL serum levels when compared to healthy subjects. No differences were observed between patients with RA and PsA.

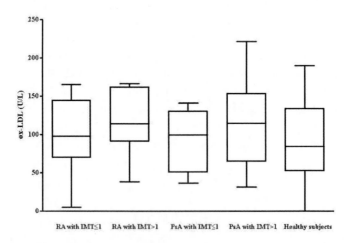

Figure 2. Box plot graphs showing oxidized LDL (ox-LDL) concentrations in serum samples from patients with rheumatoid arthritis (RA) and with psoriatic arthritis (PsA) divided according to the IMT value obtained by Echo-color Doppler images, and in serum samples from healthy subjects. Patients with RA and PsA showing an IMT >1 had higher levels of ox-LDL when compared to patients with IMT ≤1 and to healthy subjects.

When patients with RA and PsA were divided according to the IMT value obtained by Echo-color Doppler images, patients with IMT >1 showed higher levels of ox-LDL compared to patients with IMT ≤1 and to healthy subjects (Figure 2).

Serum NO Levels in RA and PsA Patients

Patients with RA and PsA showed lower NO levels in serum compared to healthy subjects (Figure 3). The difference resulted statistically significant for PsA (PsA, P = 0.0155; RA, P = 0.0655). In patients with RA and particularly with PsA, divided according to the IMT value by Echo-color Doppler images, NO levels were lower in patients with IMT >1 compared to patients with IMT ≤1 and to healthy subjects (Figure 4).

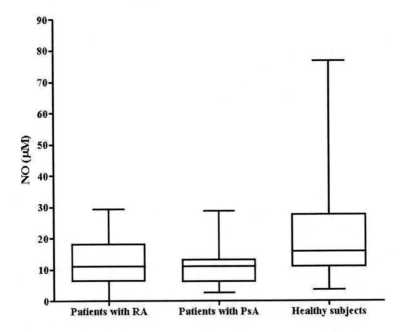

Figure 3. Box plot graphs showing nitric oxide (NO) concentrations in serum samples from the 19 patients with rheumatoid arthritis (RA), the 20 patients with psoriatic arthritis (PsA) and the 20 healthy subjects. Patients with RA and PsA showed lower NO serum levels when compared to healthy subjects. The difference resulted statistically significant for PsA (PsA, P =0.0155; RA, P = 0.0655).

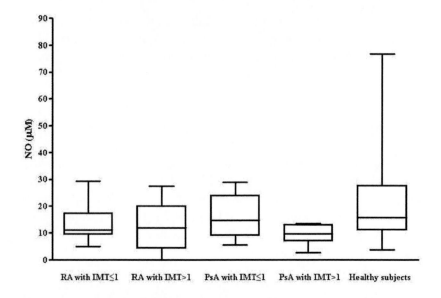

Figure 4. Box plot graphs showing nitric oxide (NO) concentrations in serum samples from patients with rheumatoid arthritis (RA) and with psoriatic arthritis (PsA) divided according to the IMT value obtained by Echo-color Doppler images, and in serum samples from healthy subjects. Patients with RA and PsA showing an IMT >1 had lower levels of NO when compared to patients with IMT ≤1 and to healthy subjects.

Association of Serum Ox-LDL and NO Levels with Baseline Characteristics of Patients

It is well known that there is a correlation among baseline clinical characteristics of patients and that these characteristics can be associated also to disease presentation. Analysis of association between risk factors and the autoimmune disease showed a significantly higher mean value of ESR and HDL-cholesterol in patients with AR than in patients with PsA (P = 0.01 and P = 0.02) (Table). In contrast the triglycerides value was significantly higher in patients with PsA than in patients with RA (P = 0.0177). In patients with RA, comparative analysis of risk factors with serum ox-LDL and NO levels showed a significant negative correlation between HDL-cholesterol and NO mean level (r = -0.6, P = 0.013) and a positive correlation near to the statistical significance between ox-LDL and cholesterol (r = 0.5, P = 0.0528). We did not find any correlation between traditional risk factors and the presence of subclinical atherosclerosis in patients with RA and PsA.

CONCLUSION

Our preliminary findings reported in this chapter indicate that serum levels of ox-LDL and NO are putative biomarkers for atherosclerosis development in patients with RA and PsA. We found that serum ox-LDL levels, higher in patients with RA and PsA than in healthy subjects, were particularly higher in patients with subclinical atherosclerosis evaluated as IMT increase by Echo-color Doppler. In contrast serum NO levels resulted lower in patients with RA and PsA than in healthy subjects, particularly in patients with an increase in the IMT value (IMT >1). Our results of a negative association between ox-LDL and NO in patients are in line with previous findings indicating that ox-LDL impairs NO signaling and endothelial function thus contributing to the pathogenesis of atherosclerosis [24]. The endothelium plays a central role in overall vascular homeostasis by regulating vasoreactivity, platelet activation, leukocyte adhesion, and smooth muscle cell proliferation and migration. Endothelial NO, an important vasoprotective molecule, is a major modulator of these effects, and impaired NO signaling with associated endothelial activation is considered an early marker of the atherogenic process. Nitric oxide is produced by the action of endothelial NO synthase (eNOS), which uses L-arginine as its substrate [25]. However, L-arginine is also a substrate for arginase, which converts L-arginine to L-ornithine and urea [26]. Thus, substrate availability to, and thereby enzymatic products of either enzyme may be influenced by the activity and substrate utilization of the other. In human aortic endothelial cells, ox-LDL stimulation increases arginase enzyme activity in a time- and dose-dependent manner [27]. Thus, ox-LDLs increase arginase activity by a sequence of regulatory events, and this increased arginase activity contributes to ox-LDL-dependent impairment of NO production.

A limitation of our study is the low number of patients that probably does not allow to reach the statistical significance between the observed differences. The low number of patients also limits the possibility to find correlation of the two biomarkers evaluated in this study with traditional risk factors for atherosclerosis or clinical features of the rheumatic disease. Of note, in our study population the only statistically significant association was the negative correlation between NO and HDL-cholesterol levels in RA. Low levels of HDL cholesterol are usually recognized as an important independent risk factor for occurrence of cardiovascular events [28]. However, Agerholm-Larsen et al. observed an association of decreased HDL cholesterol levels with a paradoxical lower risk of ischemic heart disease in women [29]. These data suggest the hypothesis that the strong inverse association between HDL cholesterol concentrations and the occurrence of cardiovascular events observed in prospective epidemiological population studies is not due to HDL cholesterol levels per se, and that individuals with low HDL cholesterol may have a reduced risk of cardiovascular event occurrence. In the light of these previous data, it is not surprising the association between decreased levels of the vasoprotective mediator NO and increased concentrations of HDL cholesterol that we observed in patients with RA.

In conclusion, our study, although very preliminary and although not establishing a causal link between ox-LDL or NO levels and accelerated atherosclerosis, suggests that ox-LDL and NO levels may be operational as markers of atherosclerotic disease in patients with RA and PsA. The detection of circulating ox-LDL and NO levels in these patients might be a useful adjunct to imaging procedures as prognostic markers for the development of atherosclerotic disease and could be useful to the clinical management of patients. Clearly these interesting possibilities await confirmation in a larger number of patients.

REFERENCES

[1]   Haugeberg G, Ørstavik RE, Kvien TK. Effects of rheumatoid arthritis on bone. *Curr. Opin. Rheumatol.* 2003;15(4):469-75.

[2]   Lourida ES, Georgiadis AN, Papavasiliou EC, Papathanasiou AI, Drosos AA, Tselepis AD. Patients with early rheumatoid arthritis exhibit elevated autoantibody titers against mildly oxidized low-density lipoprotein and exhibit decreased activity of the lipoprotein-associated phospholipase A2. *Arthritis Res. Ther.* 2007;9(1):R19.

[3]   Gabriel SE, Crowson CS, Kremers HM, Doran MF, Turesson C, O'Fallon WM, Matteson EL. Survival in rheumatoid arthritis: a population-based analysis of trends over 40 years. *Arthritis Rheum.* 2003;48:54–8.

[4]   Symmons DP. Looking back: rheumatoid arthritis – aetiology, occurrence and mortality. *Rheumatology.* 2005;44:iv14–7.

[5]   Goodson N. Coronary artery disease and rheumatoid arthritis. *Curr. Opin. Rheumatol.* 2002;14:115–20.

[6]   Van Doornum S, McColl G, Wicks I. Accelerated atherosclerosis: an extraarticular feature of rheumatoid arthritis? *Arthritis Rheum.* 2002;46:862–73.

[7]   Ritchlin C. Psoriatic disease--from skin to bone. *Nat. Clin. Pract. Rheumatol.* 2007;3:698-706.

[8]   Gonzalez-Juanatey C, Llorca J, Miranda-Filloy JA, Amigo-Diaz E, Testa A,Garcia-Porrua C, Martin J, Gonzalez-Gay MA. Endothelial dysfunction in psoriatic arthritis patients without clinically evident cardiovascular disease or classic atherosclerosis risk factors. *Arthritis Rheum.* 2007;57:287-93.

[9]   Kimhi O, Caspi D, Bornstein NM, Maharshak N, Gur A, Arbel Y, Comaneshter D, Paran D, Wigler I, Levartovsky D, Berliner S, Elkayam O. Prevalence and risk factors of atherosclerosis in patients with psoriatic arthritis. *Semin. Arthritis Rheum.* 2007;36(4):203-9.

[10] Hahn BH, Grossman J, Chen W, McMahon M. The pathogenesis of atherosclerosis in autoimmune rheumatic diseases: roles of inflammation and dyslipidemia. *J. Autoimmun.* 2007;28:69-75.

[11] Gállego J, Martínez Vila E, Muñoz R. Patients at high risk for ischemic stroke: identification and actions. *Cerebrovasc. Dis.* 2007;24 Suppl 1:49-63.

[12] Pearson TA. New tools for coronary risk assessment: what are their advantages and limitations? *Circulation.* 2002;105:886-92.

[13] Steiner G. Atherosclerosis in type 2 diabetes: a role for fibrate therapy? *Diab. Vasc. Dis. Res.* 2007;4:368-74.

[14] Juonala M, Viikari JS, Rönnemaa T, Marniemi J, Jula A, Loo BM, Raitakari OT. Associations of Dyslipidemias From Childhood to Adulthood With Carotid Intima-Media Thickness, Elasticity, and Brachial Flow-Mediated Dilatation in Adulthood. The Cardiovascular Risk in Young Finns Study. *Arterioscler. Thromb Vasc. Biol.* 2008 Feb 28; [Epub ahead of print].

[15] Michos ED, Vaidya D, Gapstur SM, Schreiner PJ, Golden SH, Wong ND, Criqui MH, Ouyang P. Sex hormones, sex hormone binding globulin, and abdominal aortic calcification in women and men in the multi-ethnic study of atherosclerosis (MESA). *Atherosclerosis.* 2008 Feb 7; [Epub ahead of print].

[16] Assayag EB, Bova I, Kesler A, Berliner S, Shapira I, Bornstein NM. Erythrocyte aggregation as an early biomarker in patients with asymptomatic carotid stenosis. *Dis. Markers.* 2008;24:33-9.

[17] de Ferranti SD, Rifai N. C-reactive protein: a nontraditional serum marker of cardiovascular risk. *Cardiovasc. Pathol.* 2007;16(1):14-21.

[18] Kabuyama Y, Kitamura T, Yamaki J, Homma MK, Kikuchi S, Homma Y. Involvement of thioredoxin reductase 1 in the regulation of redox balance and viability of rheumatoid synovial cells. *Biochem. Biophys. Res. Commun.* 2008;367:491-6.

[19] Firuzi O, Fuksa L, Spadaro C, Bousová I, Riccieri V, Spadaro A, Petrucci R, Marrosu G, Saso L. Oxidative stress parameters in different systemic rheumatic diseases. *J. Pharm. Pharmacol.* 2006;58:951-7.

[20] Spinetti G, Kraenkel N, Emanueli C, Madeddu P. Diabetes and Vessel Wall Remodeling: from Mechanistic Insights to Regenerative Therapies. *Cardiovasc. Res.* 2008 Feb 15; [Epub ahead of print].

[21] Gracia-Sancho J, Laviña B, Rodríguez-Vilarrupla A, García-Calderó H, Fernández M, Bosch J, García-Pagán JC. Increased oxidative stress in cirrhotic rat livers: A potential mechanism contributing to reduced nitric oxide bioavailability. *Hepatology.* 2007 Dec 10; [Epub ahead of print].

[22] Arnett FC, Edworthy SM, Bloch DA, McShane DJ, Fries JF and Cooper NS, Healey LA, Kaplan SR, Liang MH, Luthra HS, et al. The American Rheumatism Association 1987 revised criteria fort the classification of rheumatoid arthritis. *Arthritis Rheum.* **1988;31:**315–24.

[23] Taylor W, Gladman D, Helliwell Ph, Marchesoni A, Mease Ph, Mielants H, and the CASPAR Study Group. Classification criteria for psoriatic arthritis. Development of new criteria from a large international study. *Arthritis Rheum.* 2006;54:2665-73.

[24] Ryoo S, Lemmon CA, Soucy KG, Gupta G, White AR, Nyhan D, Shoukas A, Romer LH, Berkowitz DE. Oxidized low-density lipoprotein-dependent endothelial arginase II activation contributes to impaired nitric oxide signaling. *Circ. Res.* 2006;99:951-60.

[25] Flam BR, Eichler DC, Solomonson LP. Endothelial nitric oxide production is tightly coupled to the citrulline-NO cycle. *Nitric. Oxide.* 2007;17:115-21.

[26] Durante W, Johnson FK, Johnson RA. Arginase: a critical regulator of nitric oxide synthesis and vascular function. *Clin. Exp. Pharmacol. Physiol.* 2007;34:906-11.

[27] Ryoo S, Gupta G, Benjo A, Lim HK, Camara A, Sikka G, Lim HK, Sohi J, Santhanam L, Soucy K, Tuday E, Baraban E, Ilies M, Gerstenblith G,

Nyhan D, Shoukas A, Christianson DW, Alp NJ, Champion HC, Huso D, Berkowitz DE. Endothelial Arginase II. A Novel Target for the Treatment of Atherosclerosis. *Circ. Res.* 2008 Feb 28; [Epub ahead of print]

[28] Nash DT. Use of vascular ultrasound in clinical trials to evaluate new cardiovascular therapies. *J. Natl. Med. Assoc.* 2008;100:222-9.

[29] Agerholm-Larsen B, Tybjaerg-Hansen A, Schnohr P, Steffensen R, Nordestgaard BG. Common cholesteryl ester transfer protein mutations, decreased HDL cholesterol, and possible decreased risk of ischemic heart disease: The Copenhagen City Heart Study. *Circulation.* 2000;102:2197-203.

In: Arthritis: Types, Treatment and Prevention   ISBN 978-1-61470-719-6
Editor: Marc N. Pelt   © 2012 Nova Science Publishers, Inc.

Chapter VII

Motion Preserving Procedures for Degenerative Osteoarthritis of the Wrist due to Advanced Carpal Collapse

L. De Smet and I. Degreef*
Department of Orthopedic Surgery U.Z. Pellenberg
Weligerveld, Belgium

ABSTRACT

Arthrodesis of the wrist has been considered as the gold standard for osteoarthritis of the wrist. In 1984 Watson and Ballet [1] recognized a specific pattern of carpal collaps (SNAC), other alternatives have been proposed: the proximal row carpectomy (PRC) and the scaphoidectomy combined with a four corner arthrodesis. In this cohort of 54 patients, two motion preserving procedures were compared (26 PRC's and 28 four corner fusions). The PRC had significantly better outcome for range of motion and DASH. Grippping force was not significantly different between both procedures

* Correspondence author: Department of Orthopedic Surgery, U.Z. Pellenberg, Weligerveld, 1, B-3212, Lubbeek (Pellenberg), Belgium, Tel.: 016/338800, Fax: 016/338803, E-mail. luc.desmet@uz.kuleuven.ac.be

Keywords: wrist, arthrodesis, SLAC/SNAC, proximal row carpectomy

INTRODUCTION

A lot has been written on the degenerative osteoarthritis of the wrist due to advanced carpal collapse since the pattern has been described in 1984 by Watson & Ballet [1].

Several operative treatment options have been evocated: complete or partial arthrodesis, resection or prosthetic arthroplasty and denervation All have been reported as valuable procedures. None of the comparative series between proximal row carpectomy (PRC) and the four corner procedure could demonstrate a significant difference [2-9]. Vanhove et al in 2008 [8] confirmed this, but found a shorter perion of work incapacity for PRC compared to the four corner arthrodesis

The purpose of this paper is to compare the clinical outcome for four corner arthrodesis (4CA) and for PRC.

MATERIAL AND METHODS

Patients

We reviewed all patients who were treated for degenerative osteoarthritis of the wrist due to advanced carpal collapse: scapholunate advanced collapse (SLAC) and scaphoid non-union advanced collapse (SNAC). Fifthy four patients with 54 involved wrist could be retrieved: 26 with a PRC and 28 with a 4CA. There were 43 men and 11 women with a mean age of 52 years (range 28 to 74 y). The right side was involved 32 times, the left 22 times. There were 17 SNAC wrists and 37 SLAC wrists. There were no significant differences concerning age, gender distribution, pathology and involved sides between the patients into the two groups (Table 1). Minimum follow up was 12 months (range 12 – 72).

The PRC group consisted of 26 patients, 4 women, 22 males with a mean age of 48 years (SD 13.6), 14 right wrists, 12 left wrists; 9 for a SNAC (scaphoid nonunion advanced collaps and 17 for a SLAC (scapholunate advanced collaps) wrist, all stage 2. Seventeen wore at work (15 blue collars, 2 white collars 28 patients, 7 women, 21 men with 4CA were evaluated. The mean age was 55,2 years (range 28-74). Twenty right wrists and 8 left wrists were involved; 20 SLAC and 8 SNAC-wrists; 13 patients were at work (9 blue collars and 4 white collars).

Table 1. Summary data of the cohort

	N	Mean age	Range age	M/F	SLAC/SNAC	Side L/R
PRC	26	48	28-71	22/4	17/9	12/14
4 CA	28	55	28-74	21/7	20/8	8/20

The choice of procedure was mainly determinated by the surgeons preference. PRC was judged not indicated when severe damage on the head of the capitate was radiologically visible; minor cartilaginous damage on the capitate observed during the a PRC did not change the planned interventention. The surgical procedures have been described previously by several authors.

Surgical Technique

PRC. Surgery was performed under either regional or general anesthesia. A dorsal longitudinal incisions incorporating existing scars was used. The extensor retinaculum was identified and divided over the third compartment. The EPL was mobilized radialy, the fourth compartment with the EDC tendons was mobilsed without opening it ulnarly. The wrist capsule was identified and a ligament sparing capsulotomy according to Berger et al [10] was performed. The proximal row was inspected. If no significant degenerative changes were present, the PRC procedure was performed. Sharp division of the intercarpal ligaments facilitated mobilization of the bones. The lunate was first removed, followed by the scaphoid and triquetrum. The palmar capsule and extrinsic radiocarpal ligaments were preserved. Passive flexion and extension of the hand were done in neutral and slight radial deviation to detect impingement of the trapezium against the radial styloid. Five patients required a radial styloidectomy. The capsule and extensor retinaculum were closed anatomically. Temporary pinning of the radiocarpal joint, soft-tissue interpositional arthroplasty or resection of the proximal pole of the capitate was not performed. Post-operative immobilization with cast or splint varied from 0 to 8 weeks. Thumb and finger motion were started immediately. After removing the casts, active wrist motion was started. Physiotherapy was only applied if there was a significant rigidity after 6 weeks.

4CA: The wrist was approached dorsally and the ligament sparing capsulotomy is used to explore the carpus [10]. The scaphoid was freed from adherences and removed. The articular cartilage between the lunate, capitate, triquetrum and hamate bones was removed. A K-wire in the dorsal lunate was used as a joystick to correct the dorsal intercalated segmaent instability (DISI) and temporary fixed. In twenty six cases we used the resected scaphoid as autologous bone graft. In two cases autologous crista iliaca spongious bone graft were used. Four methods of fixation were used: Herbert® screws (11 cases) (Zimmer, Warsaw, IN, USA), K-wire (5 cases), staples (once) and Spider® plate (KMI, San Diego, CA, USA). (11 times) The wrist was immobilized for 6 weeks in a below elbow cast.

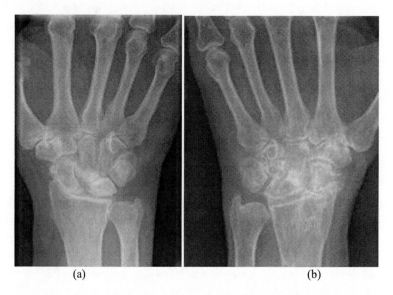

(a)   (b)

Figure 1. SLAC wrist (scapholunate advanced collpas) with good preservation of the joint between lunate and radius. (a) Stage 2 with preserved capitolunate joint. (b) stage 3 with destroyed capitolunate joint.

Evaluation

The follow-up examination was performed by independent observers not involved in the patients treatments: they asked for patients satisfaction (more than 75% satisfied with the procedure or not?). Physical examination included flexion, extension, ulnar deviation and radial deviation measured with a hand holded goniometer on both wrists and compared with preoperative values. Grip force was measured with Jamar® Dynamometer.

For evaluation of the disability, the DASH-score [11] (disability of the arm, shoulder and hand, Dutch language version [12]) and the PRWE (patient rating wrist evaluation) [13] for evaluating the outcome. The PRWE function score consists of 10 questions scores from 0 to 10 and the overall result is calculated and scored from 0 to 100. The PRWE pain score consists of the five questions (scored from 0 to 50).

All data were analyzed and compared with chi square test and students't-test and paired T-test. Significancy was set at $p < 0.05$.

RESULTS

The Results Are Summarized In Tables 2

In the PRC group 18 were fully satisfied, 8 were not. The range of motion in PRC is considerable: 64° extension (SD 11.5) and 37° flexion (SD 13.0). The gripping force, 31 kg (SD 26.8) still remains weaker than the contralateral side: on average 74%. The increase in gripping force was significant ($p = 0.025$), from 22 kg (SD 11,7) (52%) to 31kg (SD 26.8) (74%). The DASH score was 16 (SD 16.8). PRWE was 23/100 (SD 23.1) Complications were few and minor, none no secondary operations were necessary.

Table 2. a) outcome (DASH) and range of motion (ROM) (mean SD)

	Satisfaction	DASH	Extension/flexion
PRC	16/10	16 (16.8)	44° (14.7) / 37° (14.7)
4 CA	8/11	39 (30.9)	52° (12) / 32° (13)

Table 2b. Gripping force: mean (standard deviation)

	Preop force	Postop force	contralateral
PRC	22 (11.7)	31 (26.8)	42 (11.0)
4CA	24 (5.7)	24 (12.0)	36 (16.3)

(PRC = proximal row carpectomy, 4CA = four corner arthrodesis, RCA = radiocarpal arthrodesis).

Patients could regain their job at 27 weeks (SD 14.4, range 11 to 56 weeks, one was on permanent compensation) after PRC. White collar workers regained their work after 14 weeks, blue collar workers after 29 weeks.

Nineteen patients with a 4CA had no pain during everyday activities, 4 patients had moderate pain and 5 patients had frequent pain during daily activities, none had pain at rest. In the 4CA, xx were satisfied, xx0 were not.. The mean preoperative range of flexion was 36° (range 5° - 60°) (SD 13,8); at follow up it was 29° (range 10° - 60°) (SD 12,5). This difference is significant (p = 0.052) (t-test). The mean preoperative range of extension was 36° (range 5° - 65°) (SD 16,3); at follow-up it was 23° (range 0° - 58°) (SD 11.9) (p < 0.01) (paired T-test). Mean preoperative grip strength increased from 47% to 72% postoperatively (not significant p = 0.13). The mean absolute value postoperatively was 24 kg (SD 11.9). The postoperative DASH score was 39 (range 2 – 98) (SD 30,9) (Table 1). Postoperative PRWE function score was 40/100 (range 0 – 96, SD 27.8). There were 3 complications: one pin tract infection, one perforation of a screw, one neuropraxia of the radial nerve. The mean duration of working incapacity was 23 weeks (SD 17.1, range 4 to 56 weeks, 2 were on permanent compensation) Of the 9 blue collar workers: 1 was on permanent compensation, 5 regained their original job, 3 had to switch to a lighter manual job. Their mean duration of work incapacity was 29 weeks. The white collar workers were off work for 11 weeks.

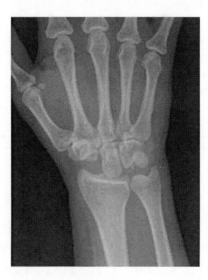

Figure 2. Status after proximal row carpectomy.

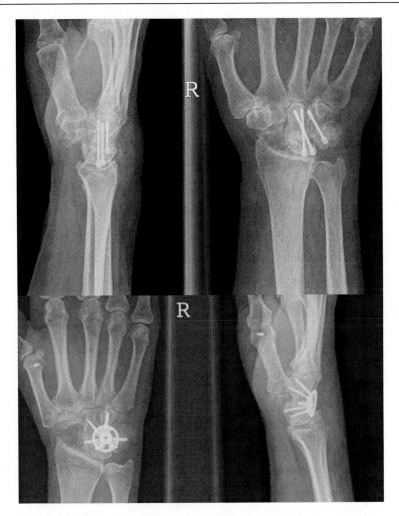

Figure 3. Status after 4 corner arthrodesis.

The DASH scores were significantly differrent in favour for the PRC (T-test, p<0.001) There was a significant correlation between the DASH score and the gripping force at follow-up: (p=0.046 with a correlation coefficient r = -0.39). However the gripping forces were not significantly different between the 2 groups (p = 0.2) Probably due to the large variation (and thereby the high standard deviation). The PRWE was significantly better in PRC compared to 4CA (t-test, p = 0.018).

The ranges of motion after PRC and 4CA were into the functional ranges. Between these 2 groups the values were significantly different (p < 0.001 for extension, p = 0.036 for flexion) (t-test) in favour of the PRC. Only in the PRC group there was a significant increase between preoperative and postoperative values (p<0.006, paired T test).

DISCUSSION

During decades and still now in numerous publications and textbooks, total wrist (radiocarpometacarpa)l arthrodesis was considered as the gold standard for unresolved wrist problems. For most insurance companies this statement is favorable since this is the "administrative" end of a sometimes long history.

The outcome of wrist arthrodesis has been studied by several authors. Their results have varied widely and the outcome probably depends on socio-economic provisions, the composition of the patient cohort and the outcome assessment used by the author(s) (14-25). However there have been more critical voices (26-29) drawing the attention to the poor patient satisfaction and the long periods of working incapacity.

The question of how much motion is needed is not fully answered. It is not clear to which extent some motion of the wrist is useful or necessary. In most impairment tables there is a linear relationship between motion and impairment. Some authors have measured the range of motion (ROM) during activities of daily life (ADL). The values were highly variable. Palmer et al (30) claimed that 5° of flexion and 30° of extension were functional ROM's, Brumfield and Champoux (31) claimed 10° of flexion and 15° of extension while the measurements of Ryu et al (32)found a much higher ROM, 60° of extension and 54° flexion. Nelson (33) approached the problem from another viewpoint: the measured to required motion to perform the ADL with or without problems, 11° of ROM resulted in a slight disability in 13 of the 125 ADL's. Adams et al [34] reproduced these simulated wrist restriction in volunteers and concluded that perceived disability was higher than measured functional loss with conventional physical tests.

In a personal study survey we concentrated on the disability rather than the impairment. In a large group of operated patients with several procedures the impact of reduced ROM (and gripping force) was correlated to the disability. There was only a weak correlation with DASH and ROM indicating that preservation of some ROM was more important than the amount of ROM. [35].

PRC converts a complex link joint system to a simple hinge joint by creating a radio-capitate articulation. The result is not physiologic and normal kinetics should not be expected, but clinical results are satisfactory in most follow-up series [36-63]. Jebson et al [48] revealed only a trend toward an increasing prevalence and degree of osteoarthritis with longer follow-up evaluation: range of postoperative motion reported in prior studies has been variable, ranging from 40% to 60% of the unaffected side. Radial deviation was consistently been the most reduced. A major criticism of PRC is weakness that is believed to be secondary to the mechanical effect of the relative tendon lengthening. A large literature review has been reported by Nagelvoort et al in 2002 [52]. They found the mean gripping force varying between 60 and 100 % of the opposite side. Trackle et al in 2003, obtained only 54% gripping force (61). In our series it was 70% (40) Only the recent articles mention the DASH score; it ranges between 9 and 36. [5,41,52,59,61]. A large series in our own department of 50 patients with a minimum follow-up of one year found a DASH score of 18 [40].

In 1984 Watson and Ballet (1) described the SLAC pattern and proposed the scaphoid replacement by a silicone spacer combined with a 4CA. Lateron, due to the ongoiing problems with silicone implants, scaphoid excision was proposed rather than replacement. Since then numerous investigators have reported favorable outcome of this procedure [64-71].

A few authors compared a PRC with a partial arthrodesis (scaphoidectomy and 4-corner arthrodesis), none of them observed significant differences [2-9]. Tomaino et al in 1994 [7] compared 15 patients with a PRC with 9 patients with a limited wrist fusion. Range of motion was significantly better after PRC; pain relief and gripping forca were only minimally different. In the same year Krakauer et al [3] found a similar result: better range of motion in PRC, gripping force was better in 4CA, but statistical signoficancy was not mentioned. Similar findings in the paper of Wyrick et al (9), all outcome measures (pain relief, range of motion an d gripping force) in favor of the PRC but none of them significant. Cohen and Kozin [2] found only minimal differences between the group of 19 patients with a PRC compared to the 19 patients with a 4CA Krimmer et al in 2000 [4] compared RCA with 4CA and found no significant difference in DASH score (33 for 4CA in 97 patients and 45 in RCA for 41 patients) and both groups were satisfied (respectively 86 and 84%). Vanhove et al [8] compared 15 patients with a PRC and 15 with a 4CA.

No differences were found except for the duration of hodpitamstay and working incapacity all in favor for the PRC. Lukas et al [5] found a beter DASH score for the 4CA (12 patients), but range of motion, force and pain relief were similar with the PRC (14 patients). For kienbock's disease, Nakamura et al [6] concluded that limited wrist fusions (13 cases) gave a better outcome than PRC (20 cases), but this pathology is completely different from the SLAC/SNAC.

The good outcome of published series of PRC could be confirmed. The loss of gripping power after PRC and the restoration of gripping power after arthrodesis has not been confirmed.

This is the first survey which demonstrates that PRC is better than partial arthrodesis, although prospective randomized investigations however are required for confirmation. The weakness of this study is its retrospective character and the possible bias in indication, but is is the question that with these results and others, a prospective randomized trial is ethically justified.

REFERENCE

[1]   Watson, K; Ballet, F. The SLAC wrsit: scapholunate advanced collapse pattern of degenerative arthritis. *J. Hand Surg.* 1984, 9A, 358-365.

[2]   Cohen, M; Kozin, S. Degenerative arthritis of the wrist: proximal row carpectomy versus scaphoid exc

[3]   Krakauer, J; Bishop, A; Cooney, W. Surgical treatment of scapholunate advanced collapse. *J. Hand Surg,* 1994, 19A, 751-759.ision and four-corner arthrodesis. *J. Hand Surg,* 2001, 26A, 94-104

[4]   Krimmer, H; Lanz, U. Der postraumatische karpale Kollaps. *Der Unfallchirurg,* 2000, 103, 260-266.

[5]   Lukas, B; Herter, F; Englert, A; Bäcker, K. Der fortgeschrittene karpale Kollpas: resektion der proximalen Handwurzelreihe oder mediokarpale Teilarthrodese? *Handchir, Mikrochir, Plast Chir,* 2003, 35, 304-309.

[6]   Nakamura, R; Horii, E; Watanabe, K; Nakao, E; Kato, H; Tsudnoda, K. Proximal row carpectomy versus limited wrist arthrodesis for advanced Kienbock's disease. *J. Hand Surg. 1998,* 23B, 741-745.

[7]   Tomaino, M; Miller, R; Cole, I; Burton, R. Scapholunate advanced collapse wrist: proximal row carpectomy or limited wrist arthrodesis with scaphoid excision. *J. Hand Surg.,* 1994; 19A: 134-142.

[8]   Vanhove, W; De Vil, J; Van Seymortier, P; Boone, B; Verdonk, R. Proximal row carpectomy versus four corner arthrodesis as a treatment for SLAC (scapholunate advanced collapse) wrist. *J.Hand Surg.*, 2008, 33E, 118-125.

[9]   Wyrick, J; Sern, P; Kiefhaber, T. Motion preserving procedures in the treatment of scapholunate advanced collapse wrist: proximal row carpectomy versus four-corner arthrodesis. *J. Hand Surg,* 1995, 20A, 965-970.

[10] Berger, RA; Bishop, AT; Bettinger, PC. New dorsal capsulotomy for the surgical exposure of the wrist. Ann Plast Surg 1995, 35, 54-59.

[11] Hudak, P; Amadio, P; Bombardier, C. Development of an upper extremity outcome measure: the DASH. *Am J Indust Med,* 1996, 29, 602-608

[12] De Smet, L; De Kezel, R; Degreef, I; Debeer, P. Responsiveness of the Dutch version of the DASH as an outcome measure for carpal tunnel syndrome. *J. Hand Surg,* 2007, 32E, 74-76.

[13] MacDermid, J; Turgeon, T; Richards, R; Beadle, M; Roth, J. Patient rating of wrist pain and disability: a reliable and valid measurement tool. Journal of Orthopaedic Trauma, 1998, 12, 577-586.

[14] Bolano, L; Green, D. Wrist arthrodesis in posttraumatic arthritis: a comparison of 2 methods. *J. Hand Surg* 1993, 18A, 786-79.

[15] Field, J; Herbert, J; Prosser, R. Total wrist fusion: a functional assessment. *J. Hand Surg* 1996, 21B, 429-43.

[16] Hastings, H; Weiss, A; Quenzer, D; Wiedeman, G; Hanington, K; Strickland, J. Arthrodesis of the wrist for post-traumatic disorders. *J. Bone Joint Surg* 1996; 78A: 897-902.

[17] Houshian, S; Schrøder, H. Wrist arthrodesis with the AO Titatnium wrist fusion plate: a consecutive series of 42 cases. *J. Hand Surg.* 2001, 26B, 355-359.

[18] Kalb, K; Ludwig, A; Tauscher, A; Landslettner, B; Wiemer, P; Krimmer, H. Behandlungergebnisse nach operativer handgelenkversteifung. *Handchir, Microchir, Plast Chir,* 1999, 31, 253-259.

[19] Leighton, R; Petrie, D. Arthrodesis of the wrist. *Can J. Surg.* 1987, 30, 115-116.

[20] O'Bierne, J; Boyer, M; Axelrod, T. Wrist arthrodesis using a dynamic compression plate. *J. Bone Joint Surg,* 1995, 77B, 700-794.

[21] Sagerman, S; Palmer, A. Wrist arthrodesis using a dynamic compression plate. *J. Hand Surg,* 1996, 21B, 437-441

[22] Sauerbier, M; Kluge, S; Bickert, B; Germann, G. Subjective and objective outcomes after total wrist arthrodesis in patients with radiocarpal arthrosis or Kienböck's disease. *Chir. Main,* 2000, 19, 223-231.

[23] Shayfer, S; Toledano, B; Ruby, L. Wrist arthrodesis, an alternative technique. *Orthopedics,* 1998, 21, 1139-1143.

[24] Weiss A; Hastings H. Wrist arthrodesis for traumatic conditions; a study of plate and local bone graft application. *J Hand Surg* 1995; 20A: 50-56.

[25] Weiss, A; Wiedemaman, G; Quenzers, D; Hanington, K; Hastings, H; Strickland, J. Upper extremity function after wrist arthrodesis. *J. Hand Surg,* 1995, 20A, 813-817.

[26] Dap, F. L'arthrodèse du poignet: alternative à la résection de la première rangée des os du carpe. *Ann. Chir Main,* 1992, 11, 285-291.

[27] De Smet, L; Truyen, J. Arthrodesis of the wrist for osteoarthritis: outcome with a minimum follow-up of 4 years. *J. Hand Surg,* 2003, 28B, 575-57

[28] Gaisne, E; Dap, F; Bour, C; Merle, M. Arthrodèse du poignet chez le travailleur manuel. *Rev. Chir. Orthop* 1991, 77, 537-544.

[29] Nagy, L; Buchler, V. Ist die panarthrodese der Goldstandard der Handgelenkchirurgie? *Handchir, Mikrochir, Plast Chir,* 1998, 30, 291-297

[30] Palmer, A; Werner, F; Murphy, D; Glisson, R. Functional wrist motion: a biomechanical study. *J. Hand Surg,* 1985, 10, 39- 46.

[31] Blumfield, R; Champoux, J. A biomechanical study of normal functional wrist motion. *Clin. Orthop,* 1984, 187, 23-25.

[32] Ryu, J; Cooney, W; Askew, L *et al.* Functional ranges of motion of the wrist joint. *J. Hand Surg.,* 1991, 202, 12-15.

[33] Nelson, DL. Functional wrist motion. *Hand Clin.,* 1997; 13(1), 83-92.

[34] Adams Impact of impaired wrist motion on hand and upper-extremity performance *J. Hand Surg [Am]* 2003 ; 28 : 898-890.

[35] De Smet L. Relationship of impairment, disability and working status after reconstructive surgery of the wrist. *Hand Surg,* 2007.

[36] Alnot, J; Bleton, R. La résection de la première rangée des os du carpe dans les séquelles des fractures du scaphoide. *Ann. Chir. Main,* 1992, 11, 269-275.

[37] Begley, B; Engber, W. Proximal row carpectomy in advanced Kienbock's disease. *J. Hand Surg.* 1994, 19A, 1016-1018.

[38] Crabbe, W. Excision of the proximal row of the carpus. *J. Bone Joint Surg,* 1964, 46B, 708-711.

[39] Culp, R; McGuigan, F; Turner, M; Lichtman, D; Osterman, A; McCarrol, H. Proximal row carpectomy: a multicenter study. *J. Hand Surg,* 1993, 18A, 19-25 .

[40] De Smet, L; Robijns, F; Degreef, I. Outcome of proximal row carpectomy. Scandinavian Journal of Plastic and Reconstructive Surgery and Hand Surgery, 2006, 40, 302-306.

[41] Didonna, M; Kiefhaber, T; Stein, P. Proximal row carpectomy: study with a minimum of ten years follow-up. *J. Bone Joint Surg* 2004, 86A, 2359-2365.

[42] Ferlic, D; Clayton, M; Mills, M. Proximal row carpectomy: review of rheumatoid and nonrheumatoid wrists. *J. Hand Surg.,* 1991, 16A, 420-424.

[43] Foucher, G; Chmiel, Z. La résection de la première rangée du carpe. A propos d'une série de 21 cas. *Rev. Chir. Orthop,* 1992, 78, 372-378.

[44] Green, D. Proximal row carpectomy. *Hand Clin,* 1987, 3, 163-168.20.

[45] Imbreglia, J; Broudy, A; Hagberg, W; McKernan, D. Proximal row carpectomy: clinical evaluation. *J. Hand Surg,* 1990, 15A, 426-430.

[46] Inglis, A; Jones, E. Proximal row carpectomy for diseases of the proximal row. *J. Bone Joint Surg.,* 1977, 59A, 460-463.

[47] Inoue, G; Miura, T. Proximal row carpectomy in perilunate dislocations and lunatomalacia. *Act Orthop Scand,* 1990, 61, 449-452.

[48] Jebson, P; Hayes, E; Engber, W. Proximal row carpectomy: a minimum 10-year follow-up study. *J. Hand Surg.,* 2003, 28A, 561-569.

[49] Jorgensen, E. Proximal row carpectomy. An end result study of twenty-two casis. *J. Bone Joint Surg.,* 1969, 51A, 1104-1111

[50] Legre, R; Sassoon, D. Etude multicentrique de 143 cas de résection de la première rangée des os du carpe. *Ann. Chir. Main,* 1992, 11, 237-263.

[51] Luchetti, R; Soragni, O; Fairplay, T. Proximal row carpectomy through a palmar approach. *J. Hand Surg.,* 1998, 23B: 406-409.

[52] Nagelvoort, R; Kon, M, Schuurman, A. Proximal row carpectomy: a worthwhile salvage procedure. *Scand J. Plast Reconstr Surg. Hand Surg.,* 2002, 36, 289-299.

[53] Neviaser, R. Proximal row carpectomy for posttraumatic disorders of the carpus. *J. Hand Surg,* 1983, 8, 301-305.

[54] Neviaser, R. On resection of the proximal row. *Clin. Orthop,* 1986, 202, 12-15.

[55] Rettig, M; Raskin, K. Long-term assessment of proximal row carpectomy for chronic perilunate dislocations. *J. Hand Surg.* 1999, 24A, 1231-1236

[56] Salomon, G; Eaton, R. Proximal row carpectomy with partial capitate resection. *J. Hand Surg.,* 1996, 21A, 2-8.

[57] Schernberg, G; Lamarque, B; Genevray, J; Gerard, Y. La résection arthroplastique de la première rangée des os du carpe. *Ann. Chir,* 1981, 35, 269-274.49.

[58] Steenwerckx, A; De Smet, L; Zachee, B; Fabry, G. Proximal row carpectomy: an alternative to wrist arthrodesis. *Act. Orthop Belg,* 1997, 63, 1-7.

[59] Streich, N; Martini, A; Daeke, W. Resektion der proximalen Handwurzelreihe bei karpalen Kollaps. *Handchir Mikrochir Plast Chir,* 2003, 35, 299-303.

[60] Tomaino, M; Delsignore, J; Burton, R. Long-term results following proximal row carpectomy. *J. Hand Surg,* 1994, 19A, 694-703.

[61] Tränkle, M; Sauerbier, M; Blum, K; Bickert, B; Germann, G. Die Entfernung der proximalen Handwurzelreihe als bewegungserhaltender Eingriff beim karpalen Kollpas. *Unfallchirurg,* 2003, 106, 1010-1015.

[62] Voche, Ph, Merle, M. L'arthrodèse des 4 os du poignet. *Rev. Chir Orthop,* 1993, 79, 456-463.

[63] Welby, F; Alnot, J. La résection de la première rangée du carpe: poignet post-traumatique et maladie de Kienbock. *Chir Main,* 2003, 22, 148-153.

[64] Ashmead, D; Watson, K; Damon, C; Herber, S; Paly, W. Scapholunate advanced collpase wrist salvage. *J. Hand Surg,* 1994, 19A, 741-750.

[65] Bertrand, M; Coulet, B; Chammas, M; Rigout, C ; Allieu, Y. L'arthrodèse des quatre os du poignet. *Rev. Chir. Orthop,* 2002, 88, 286-292.5.

[66] Dagregorio, G; Saint Cast, Y; Fouque, P. L'influence de l'angle de fusion capitolunaire sur le résultat fonctionnel de l'intervention de Watson réalisée dans 58 cas de collapsus carpiens avancés. *La Main,* 1998, 3, 363-373.

[67] Garcia-Lopez, A; Perez-Ubeda, J; Marco, F; Molina, M; Lopez-Duran, L. A modified technique for four-bone fusion for advanced carpal collapse (SLAC/SNAC wrist). *J. Hand Surg.,* 2001, 26B, 352-354.

[68] Gill, D; Ireland, D. Limmited wrist arthrodesis for the salvage of SLAC wrist. *J. Hand Surg,* 1997, 22B, 461- 465.

[69] .Kadji, O; Duteille, F; Dautel, G; Merle, M. Arthrodèse carpiene des quatre os versus arthrodèse capitolunaire. A propos de 40 patients. *Chir Main,* 2002, 21, 5-12.

[70] Kirschenbaum, D; Schnieder, L; Kirkpatrick, W; Adams, D; Cody, R. Scaphoid excision and capitolunate arthrodesis for radioscaphoid arthritis. *J. Hand Surg,* 1993; 18A, 780-785.

[71] Sauerbier, M; Trankle, M.; Linsner, G; Bickert, B; Germann, G. Midcarpal arthrodesis with scaphoid excision and interposition bone graft in the treatment of advanced carpal collapse (SLAC/SNAC wrist): operative technique and outcome assessment. *J. Hand Surg,* 2000, 25B, 341-345.

Index

B

C

E

F

Q

R

T